NUTRITION AND MENTAL FUNCTIONS

ADVANCES IN BEHAVIORAL BIOLOGY

NUTRITION AND MENTAL FUNCTIONS

Edited by

GEORGE SERBAN

New York University Medical Center
New York, New York

Foreword by
Jean Mayer

Harvard School of Public Health
Boston, Massachusetts

Springer Science+Business Media, LLC

Library of Congress Cataloging in Publication Data

Main entry under title:

Nutrition and mental functions.

(Advances in behavioral biology; v. 14)
Includes bibliographical references and index.
1. Nutrition disorders in children—Congresses. 2. Intellect—Nutritional aspects—
Congresses. I. Serban, George, 1926—   ed. II. Kittay Scientific Foundation.
[DNLM: 1. Mental processes—Congresses. 2. Nutrition—Congresses. 3. Nutrition
disorders—Complications—Congresses.   W3 AD215 v. 14 1973 / QU145 N971 1973]
RJ399.N8N87   618.9'23'9   74-28371
ISBN 978-1-4684-3077-6   ISBN 978-1-4684-3075-2 (eBook)
DOI 10.1007/978-1-4684-3075-2

Proceedings of a symposium of The Kittay Scientific Foundation
held March 29-30, 1973

Manuscripts prepared by Arlyne Zimmermann,
Director of Communications, Kittay Scientific Foundation

© Springer Science+Business Media New York 1975
Originally published by Plenum Press, New York 1975
Softcover reprint of the hardcover 1st edition 1975

This book is dedicated to researchers in the field of nutrition, who, through their perseverance, ingenuity, and dedication have advanced our knowledge on the importance of nutrition as it relates to mental functioning.

Among these scientists, mention should be made of the late Dr. Herbert G. Birch, whose premature death represents a loss which all scientists share.

FOREWORD

Not unlike other sciences--physics and biochemistry are good examples--the science of nutrition developed in this century in a manner which combined the rapid accumulation of important and useful facts with oversimplified concepts. In fact, the nutritionist--I believe more than any other type of biologist--ignored other sciences in the design of his experiments. While biochemistry and pathology were called in to analyze the effects of deficiencies, considerations of factors usually studied by the behavioral sciences, and even physiology, were omitted in the design and in the observations of experiments. The diets provided the animals were usually powdered and insipid, with the only nutritional parameter determined weight change (equated with "growth"). At best, intakes were sometimes measured. The animals were caged, illumination and temperature were constant, and no measurement of function was conducted. (It may be added that, in equally schematic experiments, behaviorists used food as reward in operant conditioning with similarly blissful ignorance and neglect of, in this case, nutritional and even physiological factors.)

In man, pellagra with its associated "dementia" (the four D's of pellagra, classically, were diarrhea, dermatitis, dementia, and--eventually--death) stood as the sole proof of the interaction of the nutritional and the psychological. Early descriptions of kwashiorkor and marasmus, the extreme forms of protein-calorie malnutrition, put all the emphasis on the somatic aspects, hardly mentioning the psychological and sociological contexts in which the syndromes developed. As in the early days of the bacteriological era, disease was thought to be determined solely by the presence or absence of the biological agent "responsible" for the disease. In this case the genesis of nutritional disease was equated with the dietary deficiency of a single "limiting" essential nutrient.

The description of sequelae of nutritional deficiencies was equally oversimplified. Obviously, a disease
like rickets, which affected hard tissues--the skeleton--
had irreversible consequences. Destruction or alteration
of tissues, such as in cancrum oris or severe xerophthal-
mia, was equally permanent and easily observed. Other
models were beriberi or scurvy, where, by contrast, the
vitamin treatment seemed to restore the individual to the
completely normal status quo ante.

Most nutritionists were therefore little prepared
intellectually for the series of suggestive findings concerning nutrition and mental development which has been
the highlight of nutritional research in the past decade:
the discovery that there are irreversible gaps in mental
development not correlated with obvious permanent somatic
lesions which follow acute malnutrition during the development of the young infant. Furthermore, not only are existing somatic instruments--physical examination, the
scale, and the measuring tape--inadequate to detect such
intellectual and behavioral deficits, but some of the
current psychological instruments, bound to traditions
of Western culture, are often poorly adapted to measure
fine differences in psychological development among poor
populations. These initial discoveries have stimulated
important methodological advances, ranging from better
staining techniques for the study of fibers connecting
brain neurons to better tests for the study of cognitive
development. These, in turn, begin to give us a better
understanding of the role of nutritional factors in
allowing the child to think and function at the level
which his genetic endowment could achieve in the most
favorable possible environment. The improvement in the
quality of psychological tests may also permit study of
the lasting consequences of such melancholy "natural experiments" as the famines in Biafra, Bangladesh, or the
Sahel.

The sociological consequences of the recent findings
on nutrition and mental development are no less dramatic.
Economists have become used to the concept of "investments
in human capital," but they have always looked upon it as
something which could be introduced as needed, at various
points in the life cycle of the population under consideration. In this view, the growth of children may slow
down during a period of economic difficulties, and the
return of ample food supplies permits "catch up" growth.
The age at which formal education is initiated can vary
from, say, 4 to 10, but if sufficient educational inputs

are used later, delays can be made up. Again, in this
view, intensive adult literacy campaigns, combined with
training for specific jobs, can replace much slower and
more expensive educational processes. Nutrition and
learning can thus be, within limits, turned on and off
without lasting consequences. With the discovery that
malnutrition can cause irreversible mental deficits, this
whole reassuring structure is in shambles. What we now
find is that unless a sufficient nutritional investment
is made into each small child, no amount of later expend-
iture can make up for it. Curiously, a corollary finding
has been that an early and continuous input has to take
place in learning as well as in nutrition; if this does
not occur, the individual will be, again, permanently
limited in his mental development.

Most students of the resources-population balance
feel that the early seventies have witnessed a major
discontinuity in the history of man. From now on, only
strenuous efforts both to limit population and to produce
more food can avert a disaster of unprecedented scale.
The recent work on nutrition and mental development suggests that mortality and morbidity figures may not be a
true indication of the damage caused by rapidly spreading
malnutrition. There is the horrendous possibility that
even when major famines are averted, there will be increases in the number of children whose minds are permanently handicapped by the inadequacy of the food supply.

It is to the great credit of the Kittay Scientific
Foundation that its leaders have fully realized the
importance of the work on malnutrition and mental development. In this one conference, they have brought together most of the recognized workers in this crucial
field. Let us hope that this excellent book will serve
not only as a précis of present knowledge, but as a
solemn warning of what awaits the world if we do not act
on this knowledge.

                                                    Jean Mayer

Harvard School of Public Health

Boston, Massachusetts

CONTENTS

Discussion on Megavitamins

Conclusion

WELCOMING ADDRESS

Sol Kittay

President, Kittay Scientific Foundation

New York, N.Y.

Ladies and gentlemen, let me welcome you to this symposium of The Kittay Scientific Foundation. I am certainly impressed by this gathering of the most distinguished group of scientists in the field of nutrition and biochemical functions of the brain. There is no need to impress upon you the magnitude of nutritional problems which face mankind at this time. Magazines and newspaper presentations are constantly making us aware of the tragic results of the tight race between population growth and food productivity. You know the tragic results. What happens with human beings due to malnutrition is, in many cases, disastrous. It is therefore an urgent and a noble task for all of you to bring light to this matter, to separate facts from passionate attitudes. As long as our understanding of this problem is confused and fragmentary, it will be very hard to convince any government to adopt a sound policy for eliminating malnutrition which is supported by contradictory or unverified documentation. No government can decide social policies related to nutritional conditions of the population without solid knowledge provided, hopefully, by you. Obviously the problem could be solved independent of you by enforced population control. Yet we all know that in any socially free system, population control does not work. Other alternatives have to be found. However, their practicality will depend on the solutions which you provide. For instance, if I understand correctly, the point of intervention in a child's malnutritional state might

1

represent the whole difference between a lifetime
of mental function restricted by slow learning and
reduced motivation, or a future of normal realization.
It is particularly shocking when we see the same situation to some degree in our own country, the most
affluent society in the world. While malnutrition in
poor countries results from a lack of minimum dietary
requirements, here it is apparently caused by
nutritional ignorance. If this is the case, it is
unfortunate for our government to spend $4 billion
annually in the war against hunger while paying only
token attention to the mass educational aspects of
nutrition. As all of us are aware, the problem with
nutrition appears to present many interacting facets,
which should be clearly separated and understood
in relation to their significance for man's mental
functioning. If it is also true that particular forms
of food and vitamin deficiency create mental disorders
in the adult, then the gravity of the problem surpasses
our expectations. Some scientists are now suggesting
that vitamin deficiency might be a contributing factor
to mental illness. If their position is correct, new
avenues will open for the treatment of mental illness.
Yet this assumption should be proved beyond any shadow
of doubt before a commitment to this treatment is made.
It is the responsibility of the dedicated and talented
body of scientists gathered here at this symposium to
bring these issues into focus and attempt to find new
ways to solve them. I am very confident in the outcome of your creative endeavors. I welcome you here,
and wish you a very successful and very pleasant meeting.

INTRODUCTORY REMARKS

George Serban

Medical Director, Kittay Scientific Foundation
    and
New York University Medical Center
New York, N. Y.

It is with great interest and concern for one of the major problems of our time, the chronic subalimentation affecting an impressive part of the world population, that we have met to discuss its disquieting consequences and its working solutions. Even though specialization within science has deepened our knowledge, facilitating comprehension of various aspects of malnutrition, it has not fully clarified the problem. The focus of this symposium is to explore the intertwining aspects of environmental and genetic factors as reflected in the physical and mental development of malnourished children. It is clear by now that geneticists do not always confirm the general observation of the clinician in the field of malnutrition. To start, the issue of optimal nutrition versus maximal nutrition raises a question as to the proper amount necessary for mental development. Obviously optimal and maximal physical and mental growth need to be clearly defined in terms of malnutrition before any valid conclusions can be drawn. In this respect another problem raised by the geneticist is the relationship between individual psychological and physiological variations as compared with group variations. Animal experiments, so important for learning neurophysiological and biological reactions of the brain to malnutrition, are requested as to their applicability to the human condition. Furthermore, research with animals proves to be contradictory in this area, differing from species to species and according to experimental design. In

3

addition, the neurophysiological data resulting from
nutritional research are raising problems rather than
clarifying issues (e.g., does malnutrition affect
mental development-when inflicted at the critical
period-by limiting any further neural growth in the
brain or by affecting the synoptic organization and
dendrite proliferation?) Apparently the degree to
which the neural system is affected depends on the
duration of nutritional restriction, but this remains
to be clearly established.

        The controversy between experts in nutrition giving
priority to nutritional factors and geneticists, or other
social scientists giving priority to social and genetic
factors is quite open. Yet apparently no methodology
has yet succeeded in clearly separating the nutritional
variables from the environmental ones. There are
significant and practical concerns related to malnutrition and its effect on mental development. We
can not afford to merely debate these concerns academ-
ically. These questions are of extreme importance and
require careful consideration in search of a solution.

        Another important issue presented for reevaluation
concerns the alleged correlation between certain
vitamin deficiencies and mental illness. Some
scientists claim to have found a new method of treatment
for mental illness with specific megavitamin dosage.
The theory and research methodology appear to be highly
controversial at this time, and require closer examination from biochemical and clinical points of view before
any final clinical commitment should be made. It is a
hope that you, the most distinguished group of scientists
in the field, will try to clarify this issue by question-
ing or suggesting methodologies which will lead to a
better understanding of the facts.

        The aims of this symposium as conceptualized by the
Foundation are: (1) to examine the fundamental principles
of each area of research, as well as its methodology and
implications drawn from data analyses; (2) to integrate
these principles with other related disciplines in
identifying demonstrable concepts in order to broaden
the perspective for understanding the problem; (3) to
explore and search for new research models which will
aid in answering our questions. With these objectives
in mind, I wish you a fruitful and pleasant meeting.

INTRODUCTORY REMARKS

Morris Herman

Acting Chairman, Department of Psychiatry
New York University Medical Center
        and
Chairman, International Advisory Board
Kittay Scientific Foundation
New York, N. Y.

This is the first scientific meeting under the
sponsorship of the Kittay Scientific Foundation. I
wish to extend especially warm greetings to our board
members from the many countries of the world--
Switzerland, West Germany, Brazil, Spain, France, and
the U.S.S.R. I am particularly delighted that we are
able to come together in peaceful pursuits and work
together in the common goal of scientific achievement.
Some of the participants in this program come from
abroad also--England, Chile, Jamaica, and Mexico. To
these, as well as to our participants from the many
areas of the United States, I express gratitude for
their efforts in providing the substance without which
a conference cannot exist. The extensive efforts of
our Medical Director, Dr. George Serban, should not go
unrecognized. To deliver this first baby required
forceps, and he used them. But the conception of this
baby was made possibly only by the vision of our
President, Mr. Sol Kittay, who evidenced a strong
interest in seeking solutions to some of the problems
confronting the human condition. He saw mental health
as an important area requiring new approaches, imaginative
programs, and particularly, research penetration into
clinical practice. I trust that much of value will be
forthcoming from these conferences, which are an attempt
to bring the implementation of research ideas to clinical
practice.

Our first meeting is a pioneering event, but it is hoped that there will not develop from it the conclusion that a witty individual made in reference to Harold Wilson, who, as Prime Minister of England, was called the modern Christopher Columbus: "Yes, he was, since he started out not knowing where he was going, upon arrival did not know where he was, and on returning did not know where he had been. And he did it all on borrowed money." Although much may be expected from this conference, it is the fertilization of ideas that is really important in bringing together scientists with diverse backgrounds and interests. There is always a gap between scientific information and its application to the relief of human distress. But it is equally true that the clinician has empirically utilized substances and methods to alleviate suffering and disease before basic knowledge was available to explain the process. Cross-fertilization in a meeting between scientists and clinicians will hopefully narrow the information gap for both. Everyone knows that in the search for knowledge it is of uppermost importance to be able to ask the right questions.

BIOPHYSIOLOGICAL ASPECTS OF ANIMAL AND HUMAN BRAIN GROWTH AS RELATED TO MALNUTRITION

INTRODUCTION

Carl Pfaffmann

Vice President, Rockefeller University

New York, N.Y.

I am very honored to be asked to moderate this
first section on the biophysiological aspects of animal
and human brain growth as related to malnutrition. As
some of you know, I came to The Rockefeller University
eight years ago to help develop a program in the
behavioral sciences, a new departure for that in-
stitution. There is a certain parallel in a way with
The Kittay Foundation with its new emphasis upon mental
health or, I might say, behavioral problems in the
biomedical context. The Rockefeller University now has
several groups concerned with animal behavior and human
memory and learning to add to the basic science aspects
of medical and health science.

To help focus our enterprise, we set up
a series of three symposia on biology and behavior
with the help of the Russell Sage Foundation. Among
that series was a symposium on environmental effects.
The first paper in the book resulting from the
symposium was a paper by Professor Cravioto entitled
"Nutritional Deficiencies and Mental Performance in
Childhood." He, of course, is one of the speakers
here at our sessions along with other participants
here who were also present at our meeting. I am
looking forward to hearing more about the progress since
then from this distinguished group now under the sponsorship of The Kittay Scientific Foundation.

The important and crucial role of private
foundations is on the minds of a number of us,
I suppose all of us at this time. The perturbations in
support of health sciences at the national-federal level
has caused concern, and the shifting of emphasis and
reordering of priorities could affect in a serious way
the scientific potential to meet societal problems:
personal problems of individuals, citizens of this
country, and peoples around the world. The field of
child health and human development is an especially
crucial one, as the evidence continues to grow on the
significance of critical periods or crucial phases in
the life of the developing organism. We are concerned with the question of irreversibility of those
changes, and that has a very somber implication with
regard to the well-being of the individual so affected.
The support and interest of The Kittay Scientific Foundation is appreciated not only by the community of scientific workers represented here, but by the international
community and ultimately, of course, by all peoples,
who will, we hope, benefit from the increasing knowledge
in this important domain.

One of the most exciting new developments in brain
science is the increasing demonstration of the plasticity
of the brain, which, for many years, had been regarded
as a relatively fixed, indeed a preprogrammed developmental process, with programmed growth and development
of nerve cells. The evidence that there is a degree of
plasticity, demonstrable at the morphological level,
appears to be one of the most exciting recent discoveries.
I am thinking, for example, of the effect of environmental
change well demonstrated in rats in the work of Rosenzweig
and others in California. The early work was looked upon
with skepticism--the need for various controls, possible
unexpected sampling bias and other matters of this sort.
However, they persisted, and I think the work has now
been generally regarded as valid and indicative of the
differential effects of environmental stimulus-response
change.

Indeed, some of the most recent work has been more
selective than this, and has focused on the growth of
dendritic trees of various cortical neurones under the
impact of environmental influences. Selective increase
in the number of dendritic spines, as in the recent work
by Greenough, for example, shows very clearly that nerve
cells are plastic and that associated with this kind of
plasticity from environmental influences, is a

similar change in development that has been known
to result from the influence of nutritional effects. It
is not simply the gross characteristic of these neural
changes that is important, but rather the subtlety of
these changes, both from the environmental and from biochemical and nutritional sources. So the scientific
task has changed somewhat since the time of the
Rockefeller University symposium to which I referred.

We at that time were at the stage of trying
to demonstrate or establish the fact that indeed there
was an influence from nutritional and other environmental
sources. Now I think the evidence is quite clear that
this is the case, and we now require the details of this
process. What are the time intervals at which this
effect may occur? Undoubtedly, there are differences
due to various factors, but it is not a question of
growth or failure of growth but rather that specifics
of these factors still need to be elucidated. For
example: are there selective influences of different
protein deficiencies or various hormonal changes?

So, this particular meeting is timely for the
speakers who will "zero-in" more precisely on such
specific questions. These are the next steps in understanding exactly how nutritional and other environmental
influences interact.

There is another theme which is emerging, and that
is the interaction between environmental and nutritional
influences in mental development or behavioral outcomes.
Speaking of human capacity, we tend to use the word
mental--but on the other hand, when we look at the data,
we find that they are very often behavioral. Some task,
some performance that we can objectively identify is
our measure of the effect. Better methodology reflects
the ever-developing sophistication of what would be
called behavioral neurosciences in this current decade,
and certainly has much promise for the future.

LONG CONTINUED MARGINAL PROTEIN-ENERGY DEFICIENCY

R. J. C. Stewart

London School of Hygiene and Tropical Medicine

London, England

Some years ago, I became convinced that early, short periods of severe malnutrition had an adverse effect on the development of the central nervous system (Platt and Stewart, 1960). It seemed probable, however, that in looking at short-term severe episodes, a much larger and more important area might be missed--that of marginal malnutrition continued for long periods or even over several generations.

Dietary requirements vary with the physiological state of the subject. A diet which is just adequate for a nonreproducing adult will be inadequate at all other stages of development. This appeared to be the situation existing in some underdeveloped communities where certain taboos and male priorities would often intensify the effect, so that children and pregnant or lactating women would be especially affected.

To test this hypothesis litters of normal, well-fed dogs were separated into two groups. At weaning group A was given a diet having a Net Dietary Protein Energy Percent (NDpE%) value of 7, which was calculated to be adequate for half-grown and adult dogs, but not for the very young or for mothers during pregnancy and lactation. The others (Group B) were given a good diet having a net dietary protein energy percent value of 10 (NDpE% = 10) which was adequate for all stages of growth and reproduction (Payne, 1965). The marginally-deficient animals

(NDpE% = 7) grew more slowly than the well-fed group, but
the growth period was extended so that, while differences
in size were considerable at 5 months of age, they had
nearly disappeared by 18 months to 2 years. This
"catch-up" is only seen in animals born of and suckled
by normal, well-fed mothers.

Pairs of litter-mate females, one on the poor- and
the other on the good-protein diet were mated at about
18 months of age to the same normal male. Gestation
times were similar for both groups so that the results
shown in Table I cannot be related to prematurity.

The average birth weights of the pups born to the
protein-deficient mothers were about 20% below those of
the well-fed group. The individual weights varied
greatly. Some, especially when the number in the litter
was small, were close to or slightly above the average
of the normal pups, but others weighed as little as
160 g. and were regarded as "small-for-dates" (SFD).
The average number of pups per litter was reduced from
5.8-4.9. By subtracting the litter weight from the
difference in weight of the mother immediately before
and after parturition, a crude assessment of the supporting tissues, amniotic fluid, placenta, blood, etc.
was obtained. On this basis, the ratio of supporting
tissue to pup was 1:1 in the well-fed group but only
0.77:1 in the deficient animals. A few bitches were
killed immediately before parturition and the pups and
placentae were weighed. The ratio of placenta to pup
was 0.22:1 in the well-nourished colony and only 0.14:1
in the marginally-deficient group, so that some degree
of placental insufficiency can be postulated.

Pups born of the deficient mothers were small with
short legs. They were as, or even more, active than
the controls, but their movements were less well-controlled. They walked with a wide-based gait and often
staggered and fell. Such incoordination of movement
was not observed in the pups of the well-fed group at
any stage, their movements being slower, more deliberate
and steady. An exacerbation of the abnormal movements
usually occurred at about 8 weeks of age, and at this
time many animals exhibited athetoid movements and even
convulsions. The full range of alterations in behavior
and movement have been described by Platt and Stewart
(1968). The exacerbation of abnormalities usually
lasted for about 12-14 days and was followed by a

TABLE I.   Effect of Protein Value of Mother's Diet on Weight Gain during Pregnancy and Weight and Number of Offspring

Protein value of mother's diet (NDpE%)	Weight gain during pregnancy (g)*	Mean weight of litter (g)	Mean weight of amniotic fluid and placenta (g)	Ratio weight amniotic fluid and placenta: litter weight	Mean number of pups per litter	Birth weight of pups (g)*	Weight of 6-week-old pups (g)*
10	3,230 ± 187 (18)	1,930 (16)	2,053 (16)	1.064	5.86 (60)	352 ± 4 (351)	2,071 ± 65 (234)
7	1,550 ± 278 (18)	1,375 (18)	1,053 (18)	0.766	4.90 (19)	280 ± 8 (91)	1,598 ± 57 (51)

Figures in parentheses indicate the number of observations.
*Mean values with their standard errors.

remarkable improvement in coordination and behavior.
Athetoid movements ceased, and it was impossible to
induce convulsions after about 3 months of age. However,
the animals were not normal. They remained short-legged,
nervous and did not join in the play activity of the
normal dogs. They were not aggressive, but were very
fearful so that normal dogs or humans attempting to play
with them might be attacked.

With the help of Dr. G. Pampiglione of the Hospital
for Sick Children in London, we were able to record
electroencephalograms of these pups. In the malnourished
group there was a reduction in the number of fast, low-
amplitude waves and an increase in the slow, high-
amplitude waves with many multifocal discharges. Although providing no clue to the basic cause, this was
one factor indicating an abnormal activity within the
brain.

Brain size was reduced (Figure 1), and the brains
of the congenitally malnourished group always fell in the
lower half or below the range of the well-fed controls.
However, when calculated relative to body weight, the
brains were large so that it was difficult to relate the
changes in behavior merely to brain size.

Histological modifications were found within the
central nervous systems of the protein-deficient dogs
and were similar to those previously described in postnatally malnourished pigs (Platt et al., 1965). They
included a relative increase in the number of neuroglial
cells, some loss of neurones and of Nissl granules from
those present, as well as increases in the number and
caliber of the astroglial fibers. Myelin degeneration
was never found, and the reduced amounts of myelin,
especially the reduction in the average thickness of
the myelin wall, was considered to be related to a
lack of deposition rather than an active resorption or
degeneration (Platt and Stewart, 1969).

It was at this time that the accommodation for
dogs was lost and the investigation had to be restarted
with rats. Diets which could be cubed and had protein
values similar to those used for the dogs were prepared
as described by Payne and Stewart (1972).

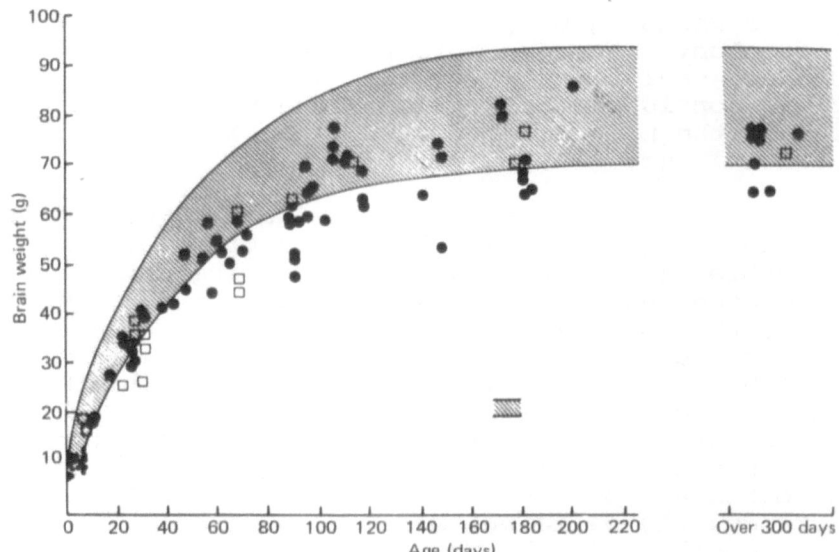

FIGURE 1. Brain weight relative to age of pups
maintained on diets of different
protein values. ▨ Range for pups born
of normal mothers and weaned onto a
good-protein diet (NDpE% = 10). ● Born
weaning on a low-protein diet, the
pups being also weaned onto a low-
protein diet (NDpE% = 7). □ Born of
mothers which were given the low-
protein diet only during gestation
and lactation, the pups being weaned
onto the low-protein diet (NDpE% = 7).

Colonies of rats developed from litter-mates have now been maintained on these diets for 12 generations. Table II shows that over this period, the marginal protein deficiency led to a reduction in litter size, total litter weight and individual birth weights. The average fall in birth weight was about 14%, but this was brought about by an abnormally large number of very small young, some weighing only 50% of the average of the well-fed colony. Any pup which, at birth, was more than two standard deviations below the mean of the well-fed colony was considered SFD. Such young were 12 times as frequent in the malnourished (29.8%) as in the well-fed colony (2.4%) (Stewart, 1973).

Many (48%) of the marginally-deficient young died in the preweaning period and the survivors grew very slowly (Table III). The slow growth during suckling can be related, at least in part, to a poor production of milk by the undersized and underdeveloped mammary glands of the deficient mothers (see Plate XI, Platt et al., 1964). Certainly, fostering the malnourished newborn to a well-fed dam led to a great improvement in the rate of growth (Table IV). After weaning, when unlimited supplies of the low-protein diet were available, growth continued to be slow (Table III) so that at 12 weeks of age, the deficient males weighed only 44%, and had body lengths only 77% as great as the controls. Between 12-24 weeks of age the absolute gains in weight were approximately the same for the two groups of males, but represented a greater rate of growth for the smaller, deficient animals. Some delay in development was therefore postulated and this was supported by changes in sexual maturation times. The stock colony from which the experimental groups were developed mated and con- ceived at 8-9 weeks of age. As growth was slow in the deficient colony, mating within the experimental groups was deliberately delayed until 12 weeks, but in earlier generations they would have conceived sooner. During the first ten generations, both colonies mated and con- ceived quite readily at 12 weeks of age, but in the later generations, low-protein (Colony A) rats did not conceive before 14 or 15 weeks of age. If given the opportunity, members of Colony B (high-protein) still mated and conceived at 8 or 9 weeks of age. Opening of the vagina usually occurred between 35 and 60 days in the well-fed rats, but in the 12th generation of the marginally-malnourished group, it was delayed until 65 days and often much longer.

TABLE II. Litter Size, Litter Weight, and Individual Birth Weights—Generations 1-8

	Colony B	Colony A
	Diet of NDpE% = 10.0	Diet of NDpE% = 6.8
	Mean*	Mean*
Number in litter	9.9 ± 0.29	8.66 ± 0.23
Litter weights (g)	54.20 ± 0.21	41.09 ± 0.09
Individual birth weights (g)	5.42 ± 0.02	4.66 ± 0.02
Percentage S.F.D.	2.4	29.8

*Mean values with their standard errors.

TABLE III. Weights* at Various Ages of Male and Female Rats Maintained on Diets of Different Protein Value

| | Colony B | | Colony A | |
| | Diet NDpE% = 10 | | Diet NDpE% = 6.8 | |
	male (g)	female (g)	male (g)	female (g)
1 week**	12.0 ± 0.1 (519)		8.0 ± 0.05 (615)	
4 weeks	67 ± 0.2 (229)	63 ± 1.0 (287)	29 ± 0.74 (276)	27 ± 0.5 (322)
8 weeks	202 ± 3.1 (219)	145 ± 1.9 (272)	70 ± 2.0 (250)	63 ± 1.5 (304)
12 weeks	299 ± 3.9 (208)	192 ± 2.0 (261)	133 ± 3.4 (239)	107 ± 2.3 (278)
24 weeks	390 ± 5.0 (137)	246 ± 2.4 (183)	237 ± 5.2 (133)	166 ± 2.3 (187)

Figures in parentheses indicate the number of observations.
* Mean values with their standard errors.
**Male and female values combined at 1 week.

TABLE IV. Mean Weights (g) of Male Rats of Colony A (10th Generation) Given from Various Stages of Development a Diet of Good Protein Value

Age	Colony A untreated	Transferred at weaning	Transferred at birth (fostered)	Dam transferred when 14 days pregnant	Colony B well fed throughout
Birth	4.6		4.1	5.3	5.4
1 week	6.5		10	11	12.3
4 weeks	29		51	61	64
8 weeks	68	119	178	237	204
12 weeks	129	206	287	314	304
24 weeks	239	283	383	443	423
Sensitivity to noise	++++	++++	++	++++	+

During the first few days of life, the deficient animals were more active than the controls. Their movements were quick, jerky and their hind legs were extended. Some, when about 17 days old, developed athetoid movements. Being more active, the young left the nest earlier and more often than the controls, and as their mothers were less responsive, they were liable to be abandoned, dying in areas remote from the nest. This undoubtedly contributed to the high preweaning death rate. The mothers did not kill their pups, except when subjected to stress, and usually did not eat the young that died. Occasionally, all members of a litter were killed, the nest destroyed and the mother found in a nervous and frightened condition. These episodes usually occurred at night and have never been observed, but were thought to be related to loud and unusual noises (Stewart, 1973). For instance, several mothers behaved in this way during the night in which a bomb was detonated near the laboratory. Sounds such as thunder did not produce a similar effect. The enhanced activity continued after weaning and, if the tops of the cages were removed, rats of Colony A--in spite of their much smaller size--were more difficult to control than rats of Colony B. There was a definite difference in body shape. The heads of Colony A rats appeared to be large relative to body size, but the facial bones were small so that the heads had a domed appearance. These changes gave the animals a distinctive appearance, making the eyes look large and bulging. There was, however, no change in eye size or weight and the apparent bulbousness can be related to the smaller facial bones.

Although growth may have continued for a longer period in the deficient animals, the adults at 24 weeks of age were of low weight, had short legs and reduced body and head lengths, and some of these changes appeared to progress from generation to generation (Stewart, 1972). There were also indications that whereas the very small offspring (less than 3 g) born into the early generations usually died, they had a much greater chance of surviving in generations 10-12. Although the possibility of an improvement in the technique of the observers cannot be ignored, the change is believed to be due to an improved viability in the very small or to a change in maternal behavior.

The deficient rats were more sensitive to noise than the well-fed controls. A slight sound which caused a mild reaction, mainly of an investigative nature, among members of the well-fed colony caused the deficient specimens to jump so that all four feet left the floor at one time. After two or three applications, the well-fed animals identified and then ignored the stimulus, but the malnourished group still jumped or cowered in a corner after 20 or more stimulations. Audiogenic seizures were more easily produced in the marginally-deficient colony, but no level of stimulation was found which led to seizures in Colony A which did not also affect some members of Colony B.

Members of Colony A behaved differently from those of Colony B in many test situations. Unfortunately, it was impossible in many of these to arrange adequate control conditions. For instance, differences in muscular development rendered water mazes suspect, as did differences in skin thickness and morphology in situations using electric shocks. Digestion and carbohydrate metabolism were altered in the malnourished animals so that the degree of stimulation brought about by food deprivation or reward might be different in the two colonies.

The Lashley jumping platform, used under conditions defined by Professor Turkewitz, appeared to overcome many of these disadvantages and offered a method of differentiating between the colonies. The results of this part of the investigation will be reported by Professor Turkewitz (see page 113).

Modifications in brain size were similar to those found in malnourished pigs and dogs, the brain being slightly underweight for age, but being heavy relative to body weight. The most marked change occurred in the cerebellum which, in the 3-month-old males, attained only 82% of its normal weight and even at 24 weeks was still 12% below the normal level (Stewart, 1972).

Although the numbers of cells appeared in some areas to be reduced, there was no evidence of cell or fiber degeneration, and the smaller number of cells must be related to a reduced production. During the first few weeks of life, the cells of the cerebral cortex and basal ganglia were small due to a lack of cytoplasm, and their dendritic development was retarded. Later, at 3 or 6 months of age, the cells attained more normal sizes and dendritic mats. Neuroglial changes, although present, were less marked than in the pigs and dogs and were restricted to an increase in the numbers

of perineuronal cells. Astrocytic fiber proliferation
was not a marked feature. The most marked changes
occurred within the cerebellum. The early migration
and remigration of cells was greatly delayed, the
malnourished animals reaching the normal 15-day stage
at approximately 21 days. In older animals, the number
of both Purkinje and granular layer cells was reduced
(Stewart et al., 1974).

     These investigations confirmed that marginal
malnutrition over several generations leads to a
smaller adult size together with modifications in the
nervous, endocrine and skeletal systems (Platt and
Stewart, 1962; Platt and Stewart, 1967; Heard and
Stewart, 1971). The results have been criticized on
the basis that the poor diets and high neonatal death
rates have led to the elimination of the larger strains
and that all the modifications can be explained by
selective breeding (Birch, 1972). Clearly, these
criticisms had to be answered.

     Malnourished animals of the 10th generation were
used for rehabilitation tests. Group 1 was given the
high-protein diet from weaning (4 weeks of age), Group
2 was fostered at birth to a well-fed dam of Colony B,
and in the third group, the malnourished dams were
transferred to the good diet from day 14 of pregnancy
(Stewart et al., 1973).

     Transferring the animals at weaning led to some
improvement in size, but at 24 weeks of age, they still
weighed only 67% as much as the controls (Figure 2 and
Table IV). There was no improvement in their behavior
or sensitivity to noise, and although the group is at
present small, there are indications that visual discrimination remains similar to that of Colony A rats.

     When transferred at birth to well-fed dams,
weight was increased to 91% of the normal, the excessive
sensitivity to noise and some behavioral changes were
reduced or eliminated, and there was possibly some
improvement in visual discrimination. Clearly, this
was an effective, but not perfect treatment.

     Refeeding the mother during pregnancy led to more
dramatic changes. Birth weights were improved to
nearly normal levels (Table IV), and in some cases,
this led to difficult births and some deaths among the
small mothers. The rehabilitated mothers, whose mammary

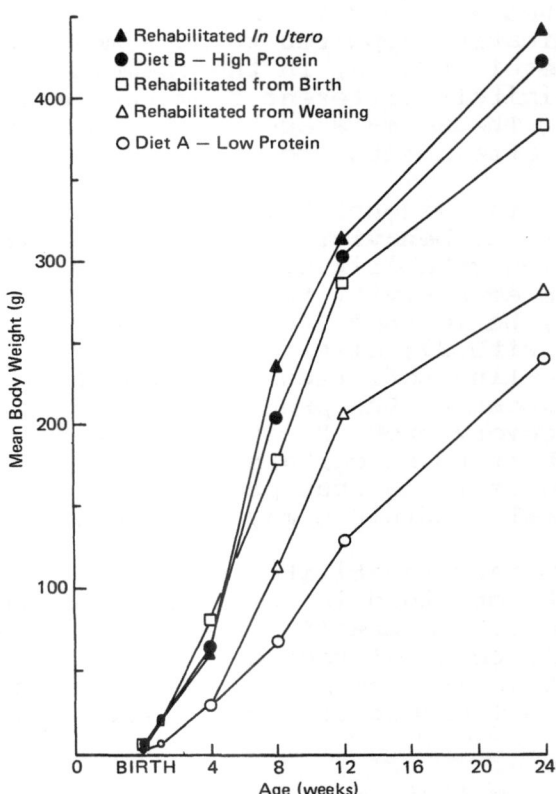

FIGURE 2.   Weight curves of animals of the 10th
generation of Colony A (low protein)
given from various stages of development a diet of good protein value
(NDpE% = 10).

glands were small, were only allowed to suckle 4 or 5
pups. In spite of this, growth during suckling was not
as great as in the control group. However, once the
young were weaned onto the good diet, they grew rapidly
(Figure 2 and Table IV), at 24 weeks attaining body
weights and lengths at least as great as the controls.
However, they were not normal, for excessive sensitivity
to noise remained as great as in the deficient group.
Visual discrimination appeared to have moved towards
the B colony level and was, in the animals at present
available, definitely different from that exhibited by
Colony A rats. The animals could not, in spite of
their physical attainments, be regarded as normal.

Thus there is evidence that various indicators of
malnutrition--size, behavior and learning--may be separated,
especially during rehabilitation. It seems probable that
changes such as sensitivity to noise and general emotional
instability may be learned from the mothers (cf. recovery
groups 1 and 3 with 2); size is controlled mainly by the
diet during suckling (cf. recovery group 1 with 2), but
also to some extent by the prenatal conditions and birth
weight (cf. recovery group 2 with 3). There are insufficient numbers to be certain of the effects of rehabilitation on learning, but present results indicate
that the prenatal conditions may be of great importance.

The preliminary rehabilitation tests indicate
that the results obtained in the investigation are not
dependant on selective breeding and that, under suitable
conditions, full physical recovery can be obtained.
Other disabilities may take a further one or more
generations. This aspect of the investigation is pro-
ceeding.

Are there any indications that findings in the
experimental rat colony can be equated with observations
from underprivileged human communities? There are
numerous reports of low average birth weights in underdeveloped areas as well as among underprivileged groups
in industrialized areas (Birch and Gussow, 1970).
Attempts have been made to relate such findings to--among
other things--maternal stature, education, home management,
and ethnic groups. The rat experiments demonstrated
that parental size may be no more than a reflection of
long-term nutritional influences, while the rapid
physical recovery (Table IV) renders genetic changes
unlikely. Udani (1963) analyzed the birth weights of
3270 children born in Bombay and found that the average

birth weights in the lower socioeconomic group was about
660 g less than that for the high socioeconomic class.
A more dramatic difference was that, whereas only 2.2%
of the upper group were born at less than 2270 g, ten
times this proportion (22%) of such small infants were
born into the lower socioeconomic group. A similar
finding was reported by Rajalakshmi and Ramakrishnan
(1969) who found that 10% of the infants born into a
low income group weighed less than 2000 g; all the
infants included in the upper income group were above
this weight.

Many children born into very low income groups die
in the neonatal period (Gordon et al., 1967) and at
post-mortem show changes similar to many of those
described in malnourished animals (see Table I, Platt
and Stewart, 1971); brain weights in particular were
found to be low for age, but heavy relative to body
weight (Brown, 1965). During malnutrition, there are
modifications in the electrical activity of the brain
and this often persists when the child is discharged
from hospital as cured (Nelson, 1959). The survivors
suffer from continuing disadvantages in nutrition,
sanitation, schooling and home conditions which may
effectively mask any "built-in" prenatal effects. Very
low birth weights have, however, been equated with later
disabilities in learning and behavior in 41% of those
born at less than 1250 g (Bacola et al., 1966) or less
than 1500 g (Lubchenco et al., 1963). Rossier (1962)
found only 22% of those born at less than 1500 g to be
at risk, and considered the disabilities to be the
sequelae of prematurity rather than prenatal growth
retardation.

It is accepted that all deficiencies in birth
weight cannot be related directly to nutrition, but
whatever the reason--for instance smoking (Butler et
al., 1972)--there is widespread evidence that even small
deficiencies in birth weight may have long-term effects.
Drillien (1969) and Wiener (1968), reporting respectively
from Edinburgh and Boston, showed that even at 12 or
more years of age the effects of low birth weight were
still apparent. Drillien (1969) showed that underweight
infants were at a disadvantage when transfers to
grammar schools were considered, stating that "low-
birth-weight children were less likely to be selected
for courses requiring a higher level of academic
competence than were heavier children from similar

types of homes" (Table V). Even when low-birth-weight
children have normal or near normal IQ scores, many have
emotional disturbances or educational difficulties
(Lubchenco et al., 1963; Drillien, 1969). These reports emphasize that small-birth-weight infants,
especially males, are at a disadvantage, irrespective
of the social class into which they are born or their
postnatal environment. This highlights the importance
of the finding that in all countries the largest
proportion of small infants is found in the lower
socioeconomic groups.

Learning and behavior deficiencies, in relation to
postnatal malnutrition, are areas of great disagreement.
Much of the difficulty might be resolved if sufficient
attention was paid to the pre- and early postnatal
developments of the subjects. It seems axiomatic that
a short period of severe malnutrition superimposed on
an already marginally-malnourished infant will have a
greater effect on mental development than a similar
insult suffered by a previously well-nourished child.
In many reports, this aspect is completely ignored, as
are differences in schooling, sanitation, infection and

TABLE V. Mean IQ Scores at 11-13 Years by Birth
Weight and Social Grade

Social grade	Birth weight (g)		
	<2000	2001-2500	>2501
1 and 2	100.0 (35)	105.7 (59)	109.9 (76)
3	90.7 (14)	97.6 (30)	100.4 (31)
4	83.7 (3)	82.6 (3)	90.9 (19)

Figures in parentheses show percentage placed in
Senior Secondary Schools. From Tables VII and VIII
of Drillien (1969).

home background, and so it is not surprising that many
findings appear to be contradictory. In a recent report,
Hertzig et al. (1972) attempted to eliminate or reduce
the effects of non-nutritional deprivation. They compared boys who had been hospitalized for severe malnutrition during the first two years of life with male
siblings closest in age and also with unrelated school
classmates matched for age and sex. The hospitalized
children had the lowest mean scores for Full Scale
Verbal and Performance IQ measures, the unrelated
classmates had the highest and the siblings had an
intermediate score. The authors discussed the somewhat lower IQ's of the sibling groups compared with the
unrelated controls and, while recognizing the importance
of other causes, regarded chronic malnutrition as a
possible explanation.

Delayed sexual maturation is also found in some
communities, especially among females, and this has
been related by Gopalan and Naidu (1972) to the general
delay in development and growth brought about by malnutrition.

Thus, there is evidence that low average birth
weights, increased numbers of very small infants, high
neonatal death rates, slow growth, delayed sexual
maturation, small brains with a modified electrical
activity, changed behavior and altered patterns of
learning occur in both underprivileged human communities
and marginally-malnourished rats. There have been claims
that some races are mentally less well equipped than
others, the evidence often being obtained from communities which have reached an equilibrium within a poor
environment. On the basis of the rat tests, it is
difficult to accept such findings, as a greatly improved
performance can be expected from these communities when
they are given an adequate diet.

REFERENCES

Bacola, E., Behrle, F. C., de Schweinitz, L., Miller,
    H. C., and Mira, M. 1966, "Perinatal and environmental
    factors in late neurogenic sequelae. (1) Infants
    having birth weights under 1500 g. (2) Infants having
    birth weights from 1500 to 2500 g," Am. J. Dis. Child.
    112: 359-374.
Birch, H. G., 1972, in: Nutrition, the Nervous System,
    and Behavior, Pan Am. Health Organ., Sci. Pub. No. 251,
    pp. 38-41.

Birch, H. G., and Gussow, J. D., 1970, Disadvantaged
  Children, Grune and Stratton, Inc., New York.
Brown, R. E., 1965, "Decreased brain weight in mal-
  nutrition and its implications," E. Afr. Med. J.
  42:584-595.
Butler, N. R., Goldstein, H., and Ross, E. M., 1972,
  "Cigarette smoking in pregnancy, its influences on
  birth weight and perinatal mortality," Brit. Med.
  J. ii:127-130.
Drillien, C. M., 1969, "School disposal and performance
  for children of different birth weights, born
  1953-1960," Arch. Dis. Childh. 44:562-570.
Gopalan, C., and Naidu, A. N., 1972, "Nutrition and
  fertility," Lancet ii:1077-1079.
Gordon, J. E., Wyon, J. B., and Ascoli, W., 1967,
  "The second year death rate in less developed
  countries," Am. J. Med. Sci. 254: 357-380.
Heard, C. R. C., and Stewart, R. J. C., 1971, "Protein-
  calorie deficiency and disorders of the endocrine
  glands," Hormones 2:40-64.
Hertzig, M. E., Birch, H. G., Richardson, S. A., and
  Tizard, J., 1972, "Intellectual levels of school
  children severely malnourished during the first
  two years of life," Pediatrics 49:814-824.
Lubchenco, L. O., Horner, F. A., Reed, L. H., Hix,
  I. E., Metcalf, D., Cohig, R., Elliott, H. C., and
  Bourg, M., 1963, "Sequelae of premature birth,"
  Am. J. Dis. Child. 106:101-115.
Nelson, G. K., 1959, "The electroencephalogram in
  kwashiorkor," Electroenceph. Clin. Neurophysiol.
  11:73-84.
Payne, P. R., 1965, "Assessment of the protein values
  of diet in relation to the growing dog," in: Canine
  and Feline Nutritional Requirements (O. Graham-Jones,
  ed.) p. 19, Pergamon Press, Oxford.
Payne, P. R., and Stewart, R. J. C., 1972, "Cubed
  diets of high and low protein values," Lab. Anim.
  6:135-140.
Platt, B. S., and Stewart, R. J. C., 1960, "The
  central nervous system of pigs on low-protein
  diets," Proc. Nutr. Soc. 19:viii.
Platt, B. S., and Stewart, R. J. C., 1962, "Trans-
  verse trabeculae and osteoporosis in bones in
  experimental protein-calorie deficiency," Brit.
  J. Nutr. 16:483-495.
Platt, B. S., and Stewart, R. J. C., 1967, "Experimental protein-calorie deficiency; histopathological
  changes in the endocrine glands of pigs," J.
  Endocrinol. 38:121-143.

Platt, B. S., and Stewart, R. J. C., 1968, "Effects of protein-calorie deficiency on dogs. (1) Reproduction, growth and behaviour." Dev. Med. Child Neurol. 10:3-24.

Platt, B. S., and Stewart, R. J. C., 1969, "Effects of protein-calorie deficiency on dogs. (2) Morphological changes in the central nervous system," Dev. Med. Child Neurol. 11:174-192.

Platt, B. S., and Stewart, R. J. C., 1971, "Reversible and irreversible effects of protein-calorie deficiency on the central nervous system of animals and man," Wld. Rev. Nutr. Diet. 13:43-85.

Platt, B. S., Heard, C. R. C., and Stewart, R. J. C., 1964, "Experimental protein-calorie deficiency," in: Mammalian Protein Metabolism, Vol. 2, Munro and Allison, eds., pp. 445-521, Academic Press, New York and London.

Platt, B. S., Pampiglione, G., and Stewart, R. J. C., 1965, "Experimental protein-calorie deficiency: Clinical, electroencephalographic and neuropathological changes in pigs," Dev. Med. Child Neurol. 7:9-26.

Rajalakshmi, R., and Ramakrishnan, C. V., 1969, "Gestation and lactation performance in relation to nutritional status," Terminal Report Am. Pl. 480, Project FG-In-224, Biochemistry Dept., Baroda University, Baroda, India.

Rossier, A., 1962, "The future of the premature infant," Dev. Med. Child Neurol. 4:483-487.

Stewart, R. J. C., 1972, "Small-for-dates offspring: an animal model," in: Nutrition, the Nervous System and Behavior, Pan Am. Health Organ. Sci. Pub. 251, pp. 33-37.

Stewart, R. J. C., 1973, "A marginally malnourished rat colony," Nutr. Rep. Int. 7:487-493.

Stewart, R. J. C., Preece, R. F., and Sheppard, H. G., 1973, "Recovery from long-term protein-energy deficiency," Proc. Nutr. Soc., 32:103A.

Stewart, R. J. C., Merat, A., and Dickerson, J. W. T., 1974, "Effects of low protein diet in mother rats on the structure of the brains of the offspring," Biol. Neonate. (in press).

Udani, P. M., 1963, "Physical growth of children in different socio-economic groups in Bombay," Ind. J. Child Hlth. 12:593-611.

Wiener, G., 1968, "Scholastic achievement at ages 12-13 of prematurely born infants," J. Spec. Educ. 2:237.

BEHAVIORAL DEFICIENCIES IN PROTEIN-DEPRIVED MONKEYS

Robert R. Zimmermann
Department of Psychology
Central Michigan University

Charles R. Geist
Department of Psychology
University of Alaska

and

David A. Strobel
Department of Psychology
University of Montana

It is a well documented fact that large numbers
of people in the world, predominantly children in
underdeveloped countries, suffer from protein-calorie
malnutrition (Behar, 1968; Coursin, 1965). Some of
the major investigations conducted with human beings
suggest that malnutrition experienced early in life
may produce a permanent alteration of the phenotypic
expression of the normal intellectual and social
development of the child (Cravioto and Robles, 1963,
1965; Stoch and Smythe, 1963). Studies concerning
severe protein-calorie malnutrition reveal profound
behavioral deficiencies in children who suffer such
a nutritional deficit before they are six months of
age (Brockman and Ricciuti, 1971; Pollitt, 1972).
Cravioto and Robles (1965) have reported deficiencies
in adaptive behavior, interpersonal social abilities,
language acquisition, and motor skills. It is
apparent, then, that children with a history of protein-
calorie malnutrition exhibit deficits in a variety of
developmental tasks when compared to adequately nourished
children.

One of the major problems in dealing with the results of studies with human subjects is that most of

the findings cannot clearly define the role of nutrition
in the formation of behavioral deficiencies. All of the
human studies are limited by economic and social variables. The human "preparation" arrives at the laboratory
as a function of a large number of chance factors such
as cultural variables, income, and nutritional
deficiencies. There have been reports which suggest
that an interaction exists among economic conditions,
family relations, intellectual opportunities, nutrition,
primary socialization practices, and weight at birth
(Cravioto, 1968; Monckeberg, 1968; Stoch and Smythe,
1968). All of these factors appear to contribute to
the protein-malnutrition syndrome in children. The
role that protein deprivation plays in the mental
development of a complex organism will probably never
be completely freed from the confounding variables in
research using only the human model.

     The animal model can function as an analog to the
human condition and provides an opportunity to control
confounding variables to a greater extent. The subhuman primate--specifically the rhesus macaque (Macaca
mulatta)--is an ideal preparation for investigating
protein-calorie malnutrition and the potential effects
on mental development generated by nutritional deficiency. Artificial diets have been developed for
maintaining the rhesus monkey separate from the mother
early in life; it breeds well and is very hearty in
captivity. Distinct phases of intellectual and
social development are transcended by the rhesus
monkey which are very similar to the phases encountered
by the human species. A considerable body of knowledge
has been assembled concerning the development of learning capacities, perception, and social behavior (Fantz,
1965; Harlow and Harlow, 1965; Zimmermann and Torrey,
1965).

     Employing animal subjects with these character-
istics permits the investigator to control dietary
programs in terms of the age of onset and the content
of the dietary regimes. Learning conditions can also
be controlled, and various social environments can be
imposed on the organism at different stages of development. The animal model is, however, limited to the
extent that mental development can be investigated.

     The natural place to search for indices of mental
development in the subhuman preparation is in the
appearance of learning abilities. A variety of

attempts have been made to study the effects of malnutrition on learning behavior in pigs and rats
(Barnes et al., 1966; Levitsky and Barnes, 1972;
Wells et al., 1972; Zimmermann and Wells, 1971). Most
of this research suggests that emotional and motivational
factors make the greatest contribution to performance
deficits on learning tasks, rather than associative or
cognitive deficits (Barnes, 1972).

Five years ago we initiated a series of experiments concerned with the effects of protein-calorie
malnutrition on the behavioral development of the
young rhesus macaque. The first subjects were 1-year-
old monkeys which were born in the laboratory. With
this pilot group of animals, the behavioral areas of
curiosity, discrimination learning, manipulation, and
social behavior were explored (Zimmermann and Strobel,
1969). Within 30 days after being provided with a diet
deficient in protein, these animals showed alterations
in curiosity, manipulation, and social behavior.
Discrimination, learning and operant conditioning did
not appear to be altered. The pilot work also indicated
that young monkeys could be maintained for many months
on a low-protein diet (Table I).

The diets were isocaloric and contained equal
amounts of the necessary vitamins to maintain the
rhesus monkey. In order to compensate for alterations
in calories induced by variations of the protein content, the carbohydrates, dextrin, and cerelose, were
adjusted accordingly. The standard low-protein diet
contained 3.5% crude casein by weight as the sole
source of dietary protein; whereas, the control or
high-protein diet contained 25% crude casein by weight.
The diets were found to be highly palatable to the
animals (Zimmermann and Geist, 1973).

Following the initial success with the 1-year-old
monkeys, the low-protein diet was introduced to monkeys
at either 120 or 210 days of age. The standard
procedure was to separate the baby monkey from the
mother at 90 days of age and house it individually in
a wire cage. The infant was fed a Prosobee formula,
and the methods described by Zimmerman (1969a) were
employed to wean the animal from the liquid formula
to a solid food diet containing 25% protein. This
procedure insured that the infant would be capable
of responding to solid food reinforcements in the
testing situation by 120 days of age.

TABLE I. Diet Composition in Grams per 100 Grams of Diet

Component	Low Protein 2% Protein	Low Protein 3.5% Protein	High Protein 25% Protein
Primex	9.00	9.00	9.00
Fat-soluble vitamins	1.00	1.00	1.00
Crude casein	2.00	3.50	25.00
Cerelose	39.70	39.00	29.00
Dextrin	39.90	39.20	27.70
Salts (HMW)	4.00	4.00	4.00
B-vitamin premix	2.00	2.00	2.00
Choline dihydrogen citrate	0.30	0.30	0.30
Ascorbic acid	0.03	0.03	0.03
Alphacel	2.00	2.00	2.00
	99.93	100.03	100.03

Vitamin Contents of the Diet

B-vitamin Premix	mg
Cerelose	2,000.0000
Thiamine hydrochloride	0.4000
Riboflavin	0.8000
Pyridoxine hydrochloride	0.4000
Calcium pantothenate	4.0000
Niacin	4.0000
Inositol	20.0000
Biotin	0.0200
Folic acid	0.2000
Vitamin B-12	0.0030
Menadione	1.0000

Fat-soluble Vitamins	mg
Mazola corn oil	1,000.0000
Vitamin A acetate	0.3100
Vitamin D (calciferol)	0.0045
Alpha tocopherol	5.0000

Blood samples were taken periodically, activity and food consumption were measured on a systematic schedule, and the animals were weighed daily. The results of these determinations have been described in detail (Geist et al., 1972) and will be summarized only briefly. There was a decrease in serum albumin and serum protein, activity was not significantly affected, food consumption was a function of the weight of the animals, and weight gain was reduced drastically. As can be seen in Figure 1, animals placed on the low-protein diet showed little weight gain over the first 40 months on the diet.

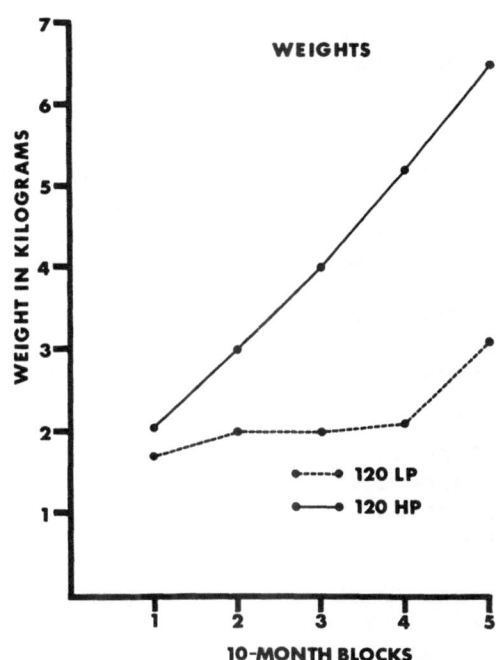

FIGURE 1. Mean weight of 120-low-protein-reared and 120-high-protein-reared monkeys at 2½ years of age.

Figure 2 presents a 2½-year-old control and an
experimental animal side by side in the social room.
Changes in serum protein occurred in the first 30 days
following the introduction of the low-protein diet
and were markedly subnormal throughout the entire
course of the deprivation (Figure 3). Blood samples
were taken every month from the 1-year-old group for
a period of 10 months, and, as can be seen, there was
no indication that the serum protein level was drifting
toward the prediet level.

    Great variation was found in the reaction of
individual animals to the low-protein diet. Some
animals lost weight on the 3.5% diet, while other
animals gained weight and had to be placed on a diet
containing 2.0% casein by weight. Approximately 5% of
the animals developed clinical symptoms of kwashiorkor
including: **"flaky-paint rash" on the body and extremi-**
ties and "moist-groin rash" of the genitals; brittle
depigmented, and sparse hair; hypoalbuminemia and
hypoproteinemia; and edema of the face and extremities.
Figure 4 shows an animal exhibiting early signs of
kwashiorkor adjacent to a control animal of equal size.
The identical experimental subject is shown two months
later in Figure 5. At this time the animal was in a
terminal state of survival, as death ensued due to lobar
pneumonia and the severely debilitated state of the
organism. This condition is now controlled by providing
the animals with additional protein at the first sign
of clinical symptoms. As a result of careful observation of the monkeys, only one low protein-reared animal
died out of 27 animals on the protein-deficient diet.

    The animals were introduced to learning tasks as
soon as they could be adapted to the test apparatus.
Adaptation took approximately one to two weeks; thus,
some animals were presented with their first learning
task when they were less than five months of age. A
significant amount of such testing was conducted in
the Wisconsin General Test Apparatus (WGTA). The
procedures followed when employing this apparatus are
shown in Figure 6. In a typical sequence, the experimenter places a reinforcement in a small food well
located on the delivery tray and covers it with an
object. After two objects are in place, the experimenter raises the opaque door separating the animal
from the experimenter and pushes the tray forward to
enable the animal to make a choice. A noncorrection

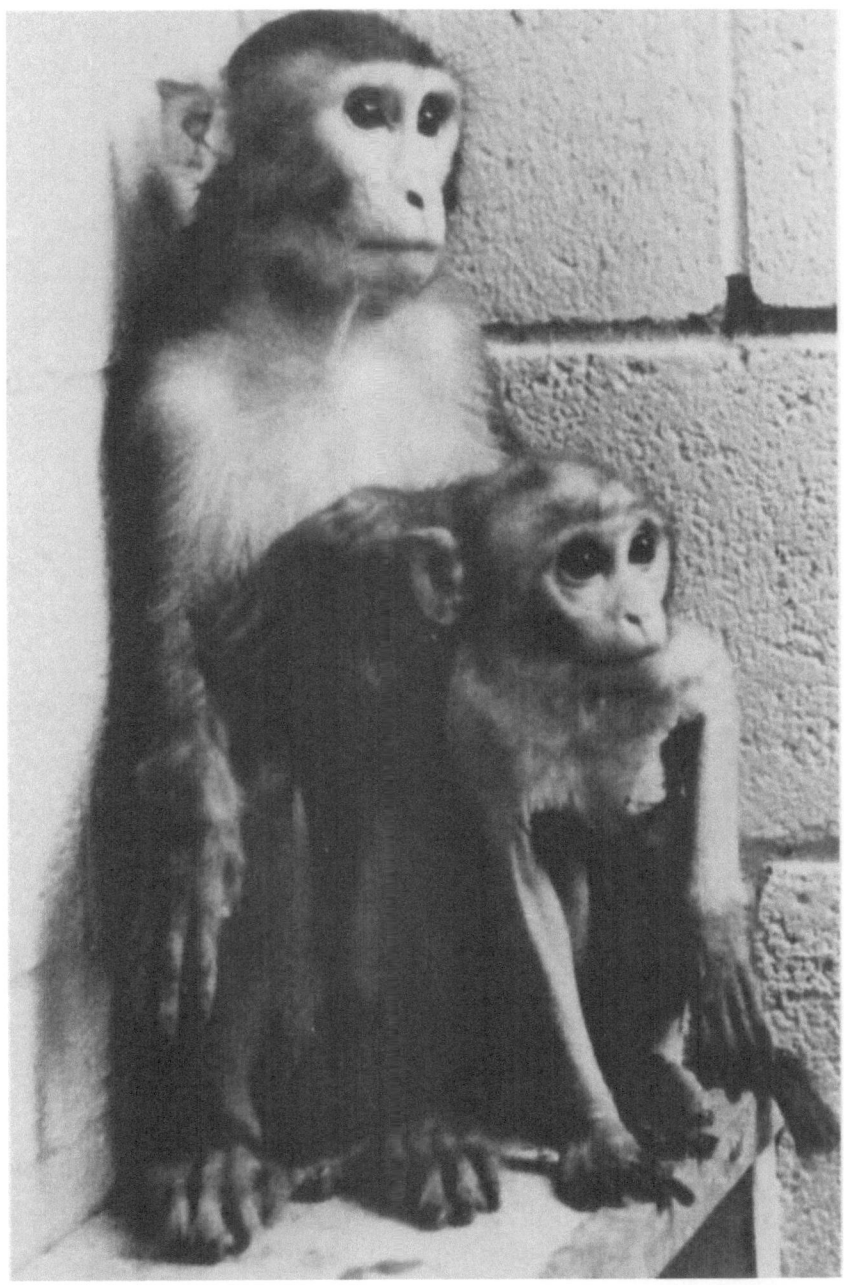

FIGURE 2. 120-low-protein-reared and 120-high-protein-reared monkeys at 2½ years of age.

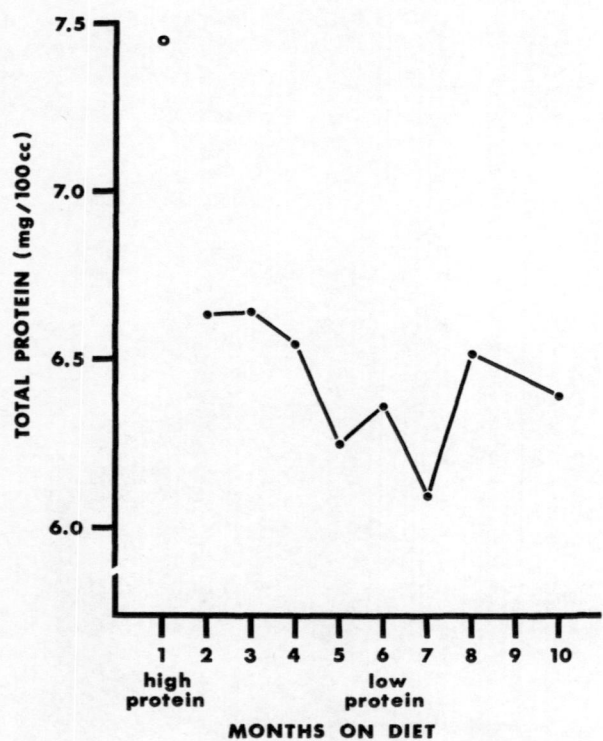

FIGURE 3. Total serum protein as measured by the
          Biuret method of the 1-year-old group,
          during 10 months on 3.5% protein diet.

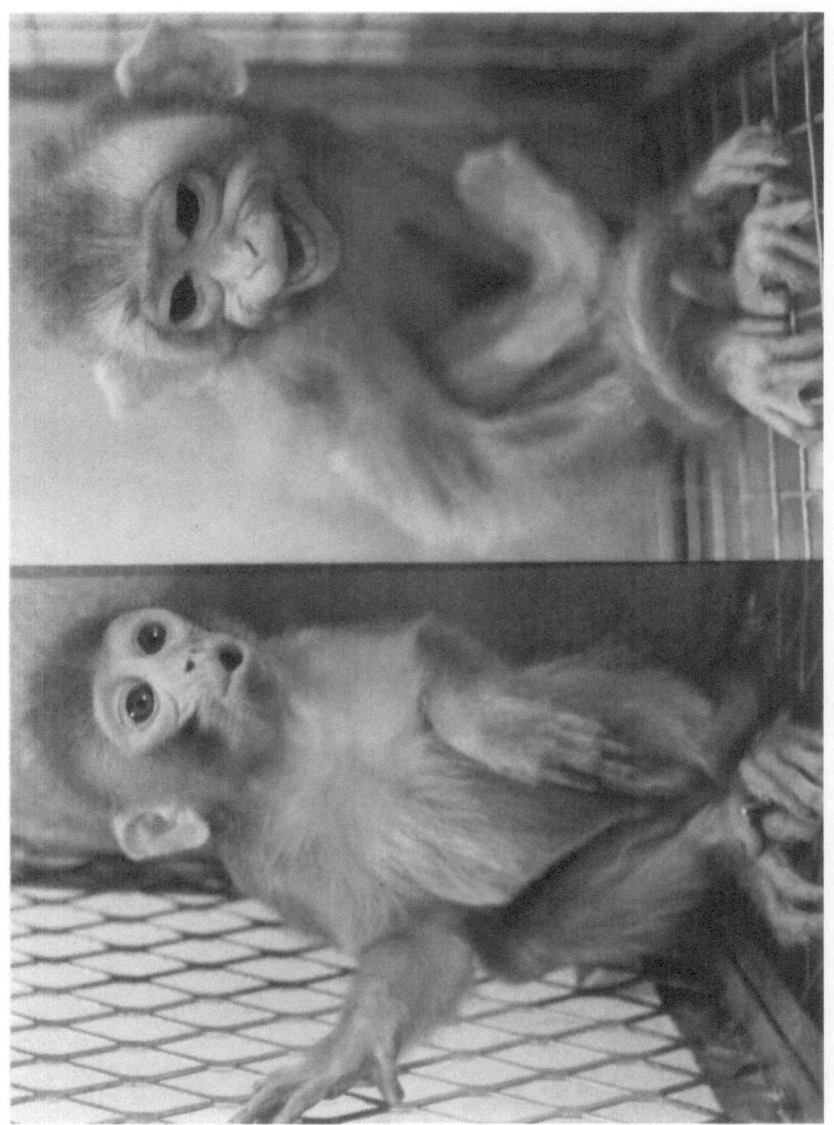

FIGURE 4. On the right, a 1½-year-old 120-low-protein-reared monkey in the early stages of kwashiorkor symptoms; on the left a 120-day-old normal monkey.

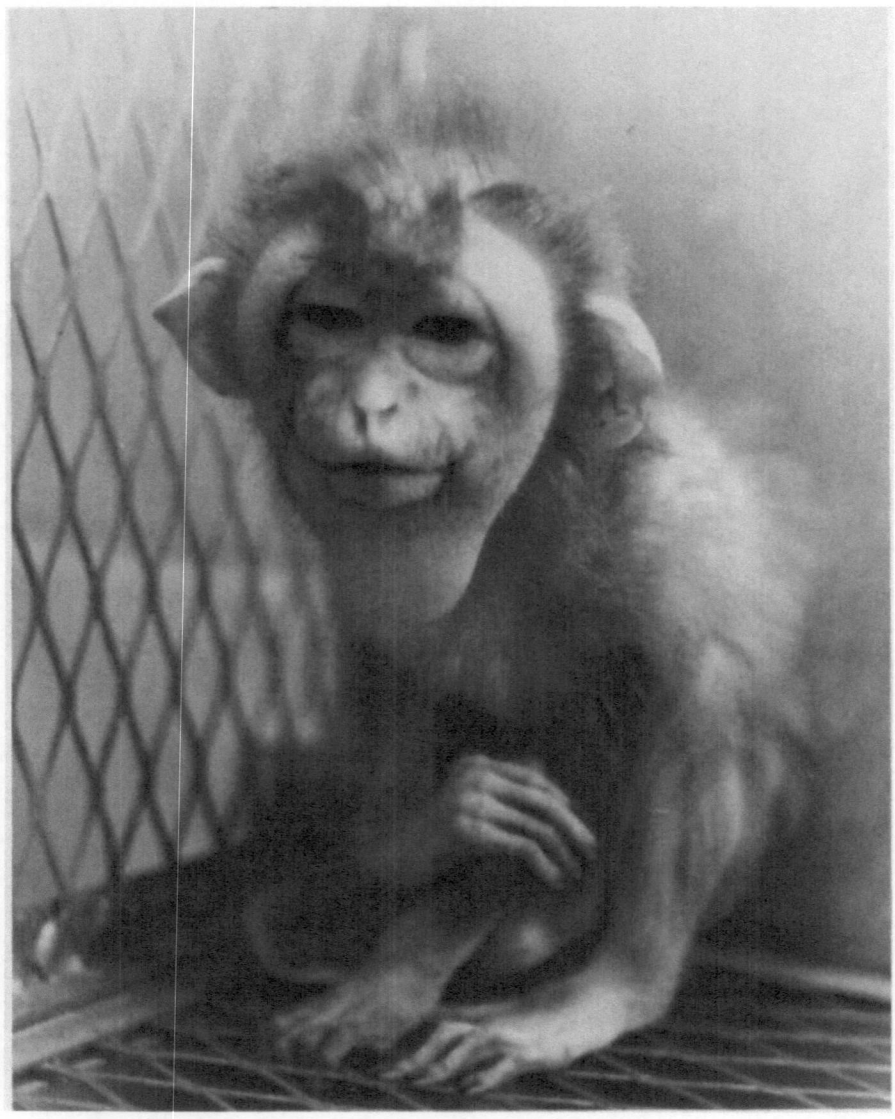

FIGURE 5. Same 1½-year-old 120-low-protein-reared
monkey (as shown in Figure 4) 2 months
later in the terminal stages of the
kwashiorkor symptoms.

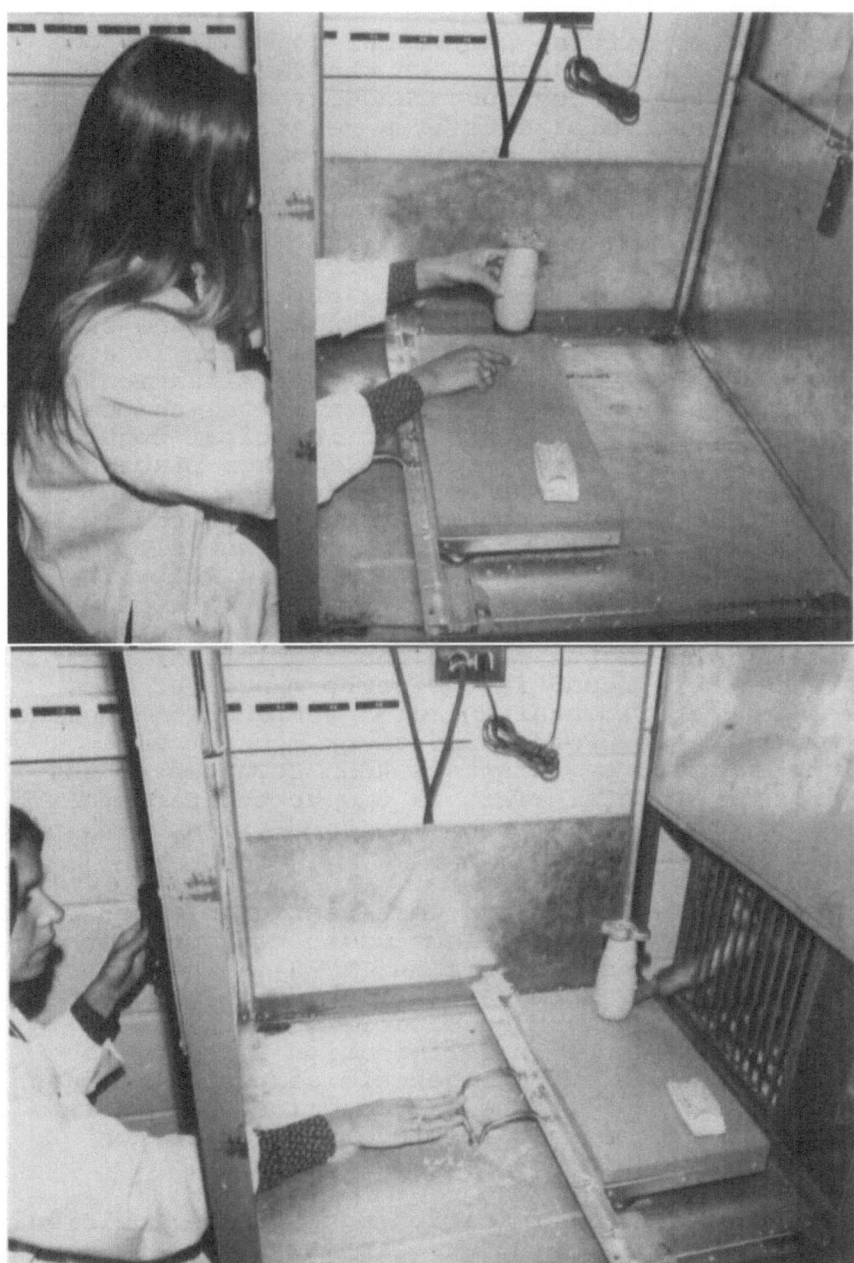

FIGURE 6. Testing object discrimination learning in the
          Wisconsin General Test Apparatus. In the upper
          picture, the experimenter baits one of the ob-
          jects. In the lower picture, the opaque screen
          separating the monkey has been raised and the
          delivery tray has been pushed forward for the
          animal to make a choice.

technique of permitting the animal to make only one response is generally used. On the first trial of each problem the monkey must randomly choose between the two alternative objects if a reinforcement is to be secured. On subsequent trials, a strategy must be learned which can be verbalized as "win-stay, lose-shift" with respect to the object if further learning is to ensue.

A variety of different types of learning tasks can be examined with the aid of the WGTA. One such paradigm is the delayed-response task which is a measure of short-term memory. In this situation, the experimenter leaves the opaque door in the up position and shows the animal which of two identical objects is to be baited with a reinforcement. After placing the reinforcement under one of the two objects, the experimenter holds the test tray out of reach of the animal for a specific period of time, generally 30-60 sec, and then pushes the tray forward to allow the animal to make a response. With delays up to 120 sec, which is probably the upper limit for delayed response in the rhesus monkey, no significant differences were found in the performances of the control and experimental animals. It should be noted, however, that the protein-deficient monkeys were slightly superior on this task when compared to the high-protein animals. This is due to the fact that the low-protein animals are more food oriented than the well-fed controls.

The 1-year-old monkeys were tested on a series of learning and reversal problems under both prediet and postdiet conditions (Zimmermann, 1973). The reversal task was selected since it has been demonstrated to differentiate the learning capacities of higher primates, which simple discrimination learning does not follow an orderly phylogenetic sequence (Rumbaugh and Pournelle, 1966). The introduction of the diet deficient in protein has absolutely no effect on either discrimination or reversal learning.

The typical discrimination task can be modified to examine other learning capacities. Learning set, or learning how to learn, can be investigated by presenting the animal with a series of hundreds of problems for a number of fixed trials, rather than demanding the animal to learn each problem to a

specified criterion, as is the procedure in most other
discrimination learning experiments. Six animals
receiving the low-protein diets, as well as the age
controls, were presented with 100 six-trial discrimination problems. After completion of the 100-problem
sequence, the subjects were given the same problems
in the same sequence for six repetitions. The performance on the 1st trial of each problem would be a
measure of long-term memory, whereas the 2nd-6th trial
would be a measure of learning-set formation (Zimmermann,
1969b). The animals reared on the low-protein diet
were consistently superior to the high-protein controls
in both 1st trial performance (memory) and trials 2-6
(learning set). Tests in food preferences indicated
that the animals maintained on the low-protein diet were
more highly motivated for food (Peregoy et al., 1972).

Because of the motivational differences between
the control and experimental animals, aversive stimulation was employed to study learning in the rhesus monkey.
In a preliminary investigation it was found that the
low-protein animals had a lower threshold for electric
shock and that they made rather gross responses to
electrical stimulation (Wise and Zimmermann, 1973).
Whereas an adequately nourished monkey, when first
shocked, directs activity toward objects in the environment, such as biting the bars of the grid floor in the
test chamber, the malnourished animals exhibited
diffuse responses, screaming and defecating at the onset
of shock. The high-protein control animals rapidly
developed different strategies for avoiding or minimizing
the shock, such as bridging across the cage to hold
themselves above the floor. This response was eliminated
by greasing the walls of the apparatus. On the contrary,
the malnourished monkeys would clutch themselves and go
into a very rigid, fetal-like position, remaining that
way until removed from the apparatus. It was impossible
to investigate learning in this condition becuase of the
aberrant behavioral responses.

In order to overcome the difficulty encountered with
aversive electrical stimulation, an apparatus was designed in which an animal would receive a short but
intense blast of compressed air if an incorrect response
was made in a two-choice discrimination problem. This
apparatus was adapted to the WGTA so that multiple
problem learning--learning-set formation--could be investigated with an aversive stimulus as the reinforcement.

In the appetative reinforcement procedure the animal
is rewarded for selecting the correct object, while in
the aversive procedure the animal receives the
negative reinforcer when a response is made to the
incorrect stimulus. Under these test conditions, both
the malnourished and normal animals developed learning
sets at the same rate. Further, the types of errors
that the monkeys made during the development of this
ability were very similar to those found in appetative
learning-set formation (Stoffer and Zimmermann, 1973).

Oddity problems are another task which can be
presented in the WGTA in order to evaluate learning
capacity in the rhesus monkey. In this situation,
two identical stimulus objects are placed on the tray
with one other object (Figure 7). The odd object is
always placed on the far left or far right of the tray
and all objects cover a food well. The high- and
low-protein groups were tested on 400 different six-
trial oddity problems. Again, no significant differences were found which would differentiate the malnourished animals from controls in learning a complex
problem. It was noted, however, that the low-protein
subjects would become very disturbed when each new
problem was first presented. They would rock back
and forth, scream, and would stay at the rear of the
test apparatus. Consequently, latency to respond to
the stimuli was much greater for the malnourished
animals than the high-protein controls. This, and
the highly emotional reaction the low-protein animals
made at the appearance of strangers to the laboratory,
led to the hypothesis that new objects or sudden
changes in the environment disturbed the ongoing
behavior of these animals.

To test the supposition that new stimuli were
disturbing to the low-protein animals, the following
experiment was designed. Both control and experimental
animals were trained in memorization of 50 different
six-trial problems until the first trial responses for
each group was 80% correct. At this time, the test
situation was altered. For half of the well-memorized
problems a new positive stimulus was introduced, while
in the other half of the problems a new negative
stimulus was introduced. The curiosity of the
developing rhesus monkey generally leads to neophilic
tendencies (response toward novel things). Thus,
adequately nourished monkeys are attracted to new stimuli.

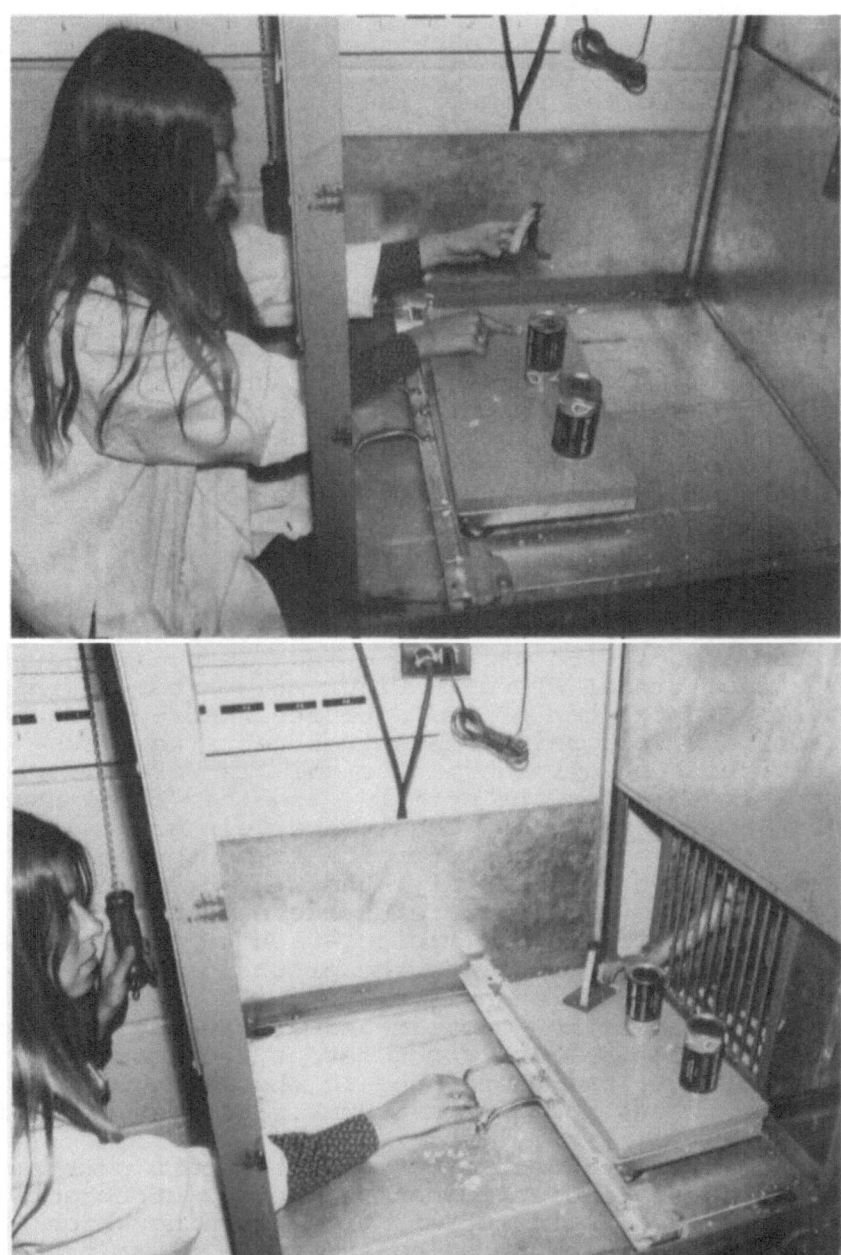

FIGURE 7. Oddity testing in the Wisconsin General Test Apparatus. Upper picture: baiting the well; lower picture: animal making response.

In this paradigm, the malnourished animals did not show
the typical reaction, but rather, showed a consistent
avoidance of the new stimuli (neophobia) in both the
positive and negative conditions. In contrast, the
high-protein controls showed significant approach responses to the novel stimuli (Zimmermann et al., 1970).

The phenomena of neophobia has been observed in a
variety of test situations other than learning. In one
such test, objects were attached to chains and sus-
pended into the cage of the monkey. The protein-
deficient animals made significantly fewer responses
to these stimuli than the control groups (Strobel and
Zimmermann, 1972). Manipulatory behavior, in general,
is depressed in the malnourished monkey, but it can be
brought to control levels by providing food reinforcement. When the food is restored, the control animals
maintain a high rate of responding, while the malnourished animals return to their prereward levels
(Aakre et al., 1973).

In another investigation, the control and malnourished groups were trained to shuttle up and down
the vertical tunnel shown in Figure 8. After learning
to shuttle to the top of the apparatus and then back to
the floor for food reinforcement, objects were sus-
pended within the cylinder. The animals were allowed
to adapt to three of the stimuli, and then three novel
objects were introduced. The low-protein groups showed
a reduction in the number of reinforcements received
in the test. To the contrary, the high-protein controls
increased in the number of reinforcements obtained.
Measures of avoidance and manipulation of the objects
also served to differentiate the groups. The high-
protein animals consistently played with the novel
stimuli, while the low-protein animals avoided contact
with the objects. Thus, a consistent neophobia, or
fear of novelty, has been found in the malnourished,
developing rhesus macaque in a number of test situations.

In an attempt to develop more difficult problems
for the monkeys to discriminate, a series of objects
were constructed for discrimination learning which
were mounted on masonite plaques (Figure 9). It has
been shown on numerous occasions that this procedure
produces stimulus-response discontiguity which makes
discrimination problems more difficult for rhesus
monkeys to learn. The high- and low-protein subjects

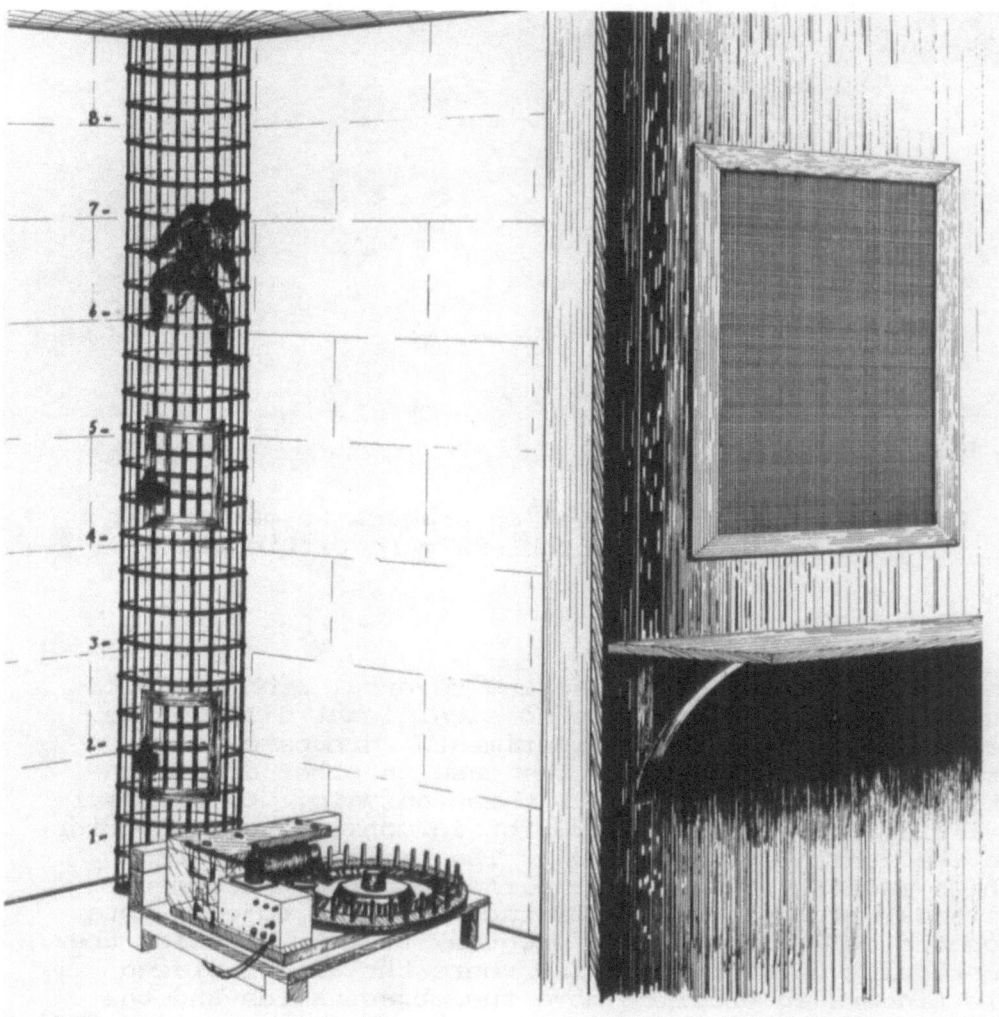

FIGURE 8. Apparatus used to study the effects of
novelty on an operant response. The monkey
is taught to climb to the top and return to
the bottom for a reward. Reinforcement
apparatus is in the lower center.

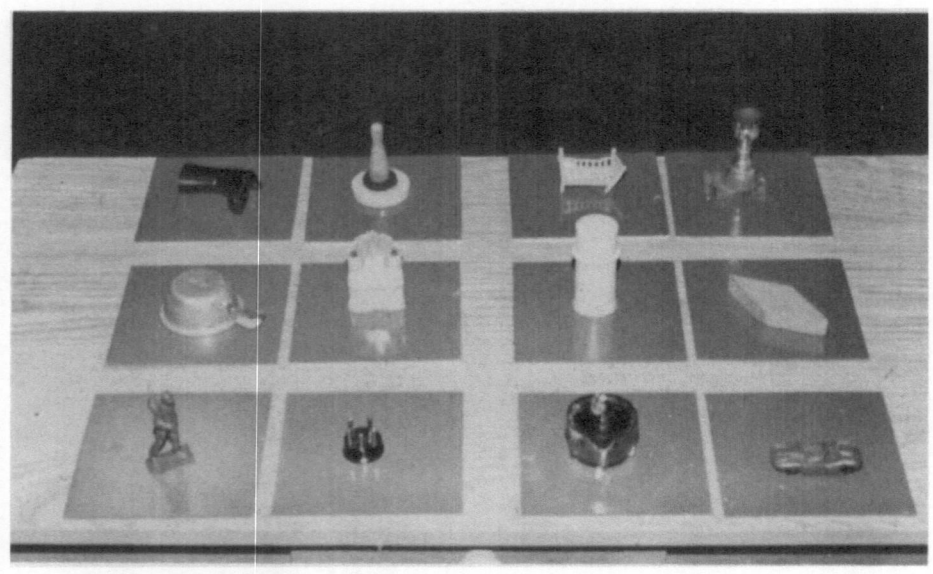

FIGURE 9. Objects mounted on plaques to make dis-
     crimination problems more difficult.

were tested on six learning and reversal problems with
these stimuli. There were no significant differences
between the control and experimental groups on
original learning, as was the case in other discrimination learning studies with these animals. On reversal
learning, however, the low-protein monkeys were inferior
to the controls (Figure 10). The significant detail
which made this experiment different from the other
reversal procedures was the fact that the objects were
mounted on 7.62 x 7.62 cm plaques, thereby breaking the
contiguity between the point where the animal placed
his fingers in order to move the object aside and the
stimulus which differentiated the pair (Zimmermann, 1973).

     To further investigate the concept that stimulus-
response discontiguity was the source of the deficiency
found in the low-protein monkeys in reversal problems,

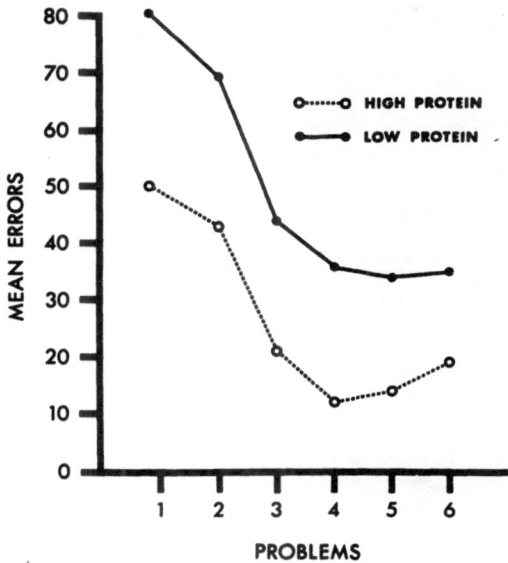

FIGURE 10. Mean errors of high- and low-protein-reared
monkeys on reversal problems using the
stimuli in Figure 9.

a set of stimuli were constructed which followed three
precepts: (1) on some of the stimuli the discriminable
cue was placed in the center of a neutral gray plaque;
(2) the discriminable cue was located on the periphery
in the remainder of the stimulus plaques; (3) the total
area of the discriminable cue on the plaques was varied
from 100% to approximately 5% of the total area of the
card. This set of stimuli is shown in Figure 11. As
the total area of the discriminable cue was reduced in
the central-cue conditions, the discontiguity between
where the animal placed his fingers in order to respond

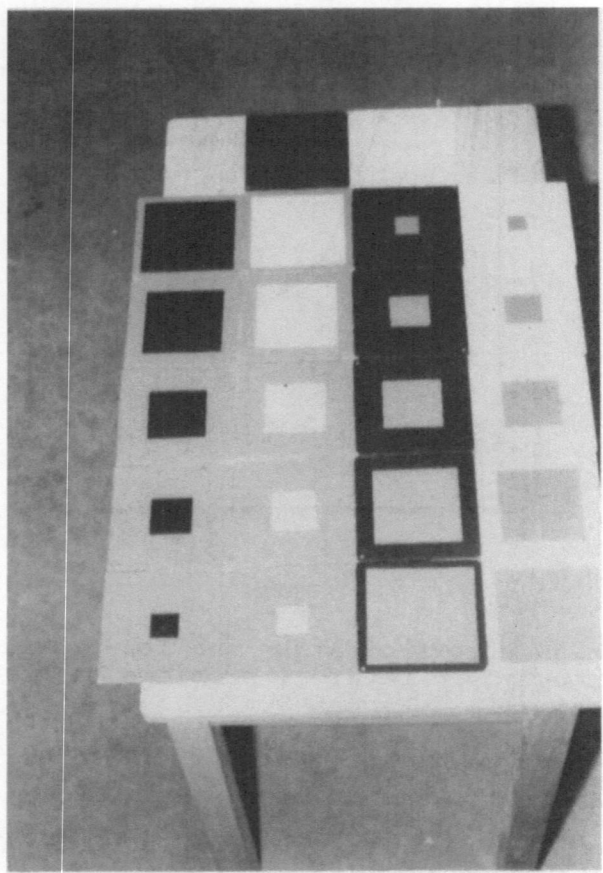

FIGURE 11. Black-white discrimination stimuli con-
          structed with cues in the center or periph-
          eral portions of the plaque and gradual
          reduction of area discriminable cue.

and the locus of the cue was increased. Figure 12
depicts a typical response to these stimuli with the
animal touching the periphery of the card. Pairs of
stimuli were introduced to the animals in a learning-
set paradigm in which six trials per problem and five
problems per day were presented in a randomized
Latin-square sequence. As found in other learning
tasks, the groups did not differ in ability to learn
the original problem. However, when placed on reversal
problems, the low-protein monkeys were inferior to

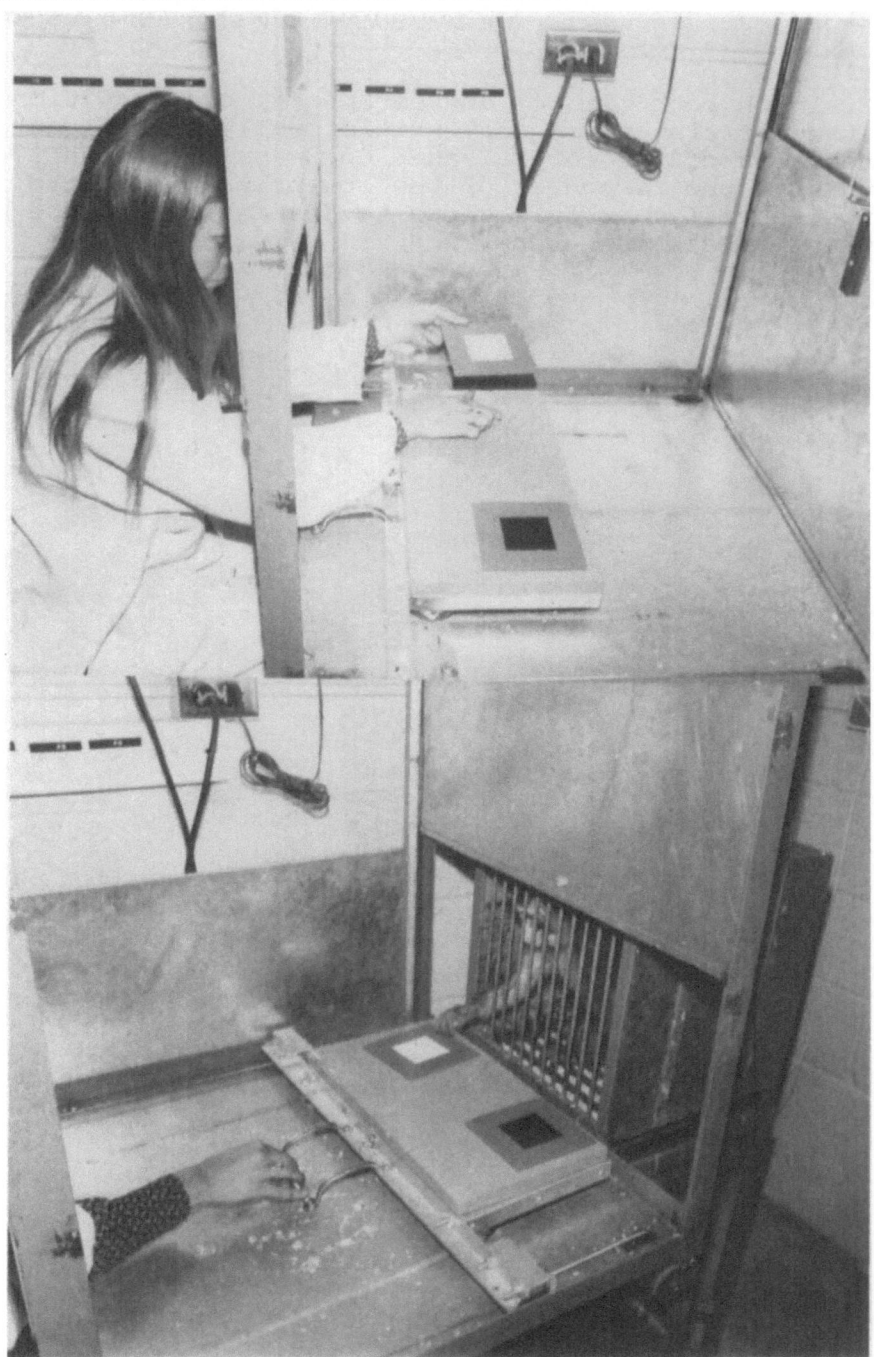

FIGURE 12. Baiting black-white stimuli with central cues
(top). Monkey responding to the stimulus
with central cue. Note the position of the
animal's fingers on the gray portion of the
stimulus (bottom).

controls on both central and peripheral cue conditions, but the difference was only statistically significant as the area of the central cues decreased. Figure 13 shows that the responses of the low-protein subjects to the central cues fell close to chance performance on the smallest cue areas.

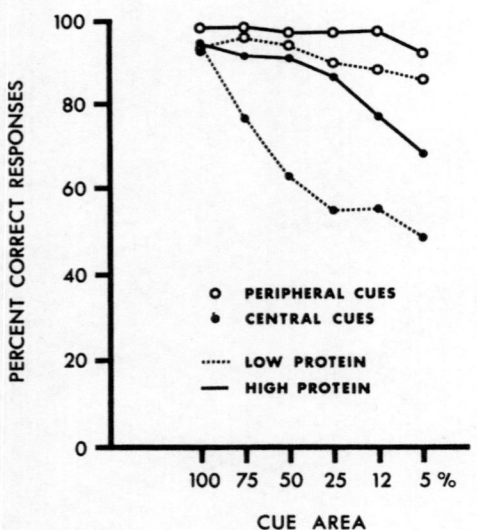

Figure 13. Performance of high- and low-protein-reared monkeys on reversal problems as a function of locus and area of discriminable cue.

Another method for presenting an animal with a
problem that separates the cue-reinforcement relations
is the conditional learning task shown in Figure 14.
The formula in this task is that when the triangle is
present in the center, the reward is hidden on the
right. When the square is present, the reinforcement
is on the left. The right-left positions were randomly
assigned to the animals in order to counter balance any
position habits that might develop for individual
animals. Seven of the nine malnourished monkeys failed
to reach a criterion of 80% correct after 2,100 trials.
All of the control subjects achieved this level of
learning in less than 1,300 trials.

In an investigation of children who had suffered
from early protein-calorie malnutrition, Klein et al.
(1969) reported that these children did not differ
from controls on discrimination learning tasks. However, malnourished children were inferior to adequately
nourished controls on tasks which required attention,
such as a rapid-tapping task and an embedded-figures
task in which the child must locate an object or
pattern in a complex stimulus. It was further noted
that the problems could be solved by the malnourished
children if the tapping sequence was slowed down or
the embedded figure originally pointed out. Thus, the
deficiency was not one of cognitive capacity, but one
of attention. The children did not seem to attend to
the critical cues which identified the embedded
figures.

The embedded-figures task could be readily
adapted to the primate-testing program in protein-
calorie malnutrition. The groups of animals were
trained to discriminate a square from a triangle until
a level of 90% correct, or better, was achieved on two
consecutive days. After learning this problem, the
animals were tested on a transfer task employing the
stimuli depicted in Figure 15. The percentage of
correct responses made to all of the stimulus pairs
in the transfer test are presented in Figure 16. The
animals maintained on the high-protein diet were
superior in the initial responses to the patterns and
showed an improvement across the 20-test trials. In
contrast, the low-protein subjects did not respond
significantly above chance to the stimuli. Therefore,
the findings reported by Klein et al. (1969) have
been confirmed in the subhuman primate.

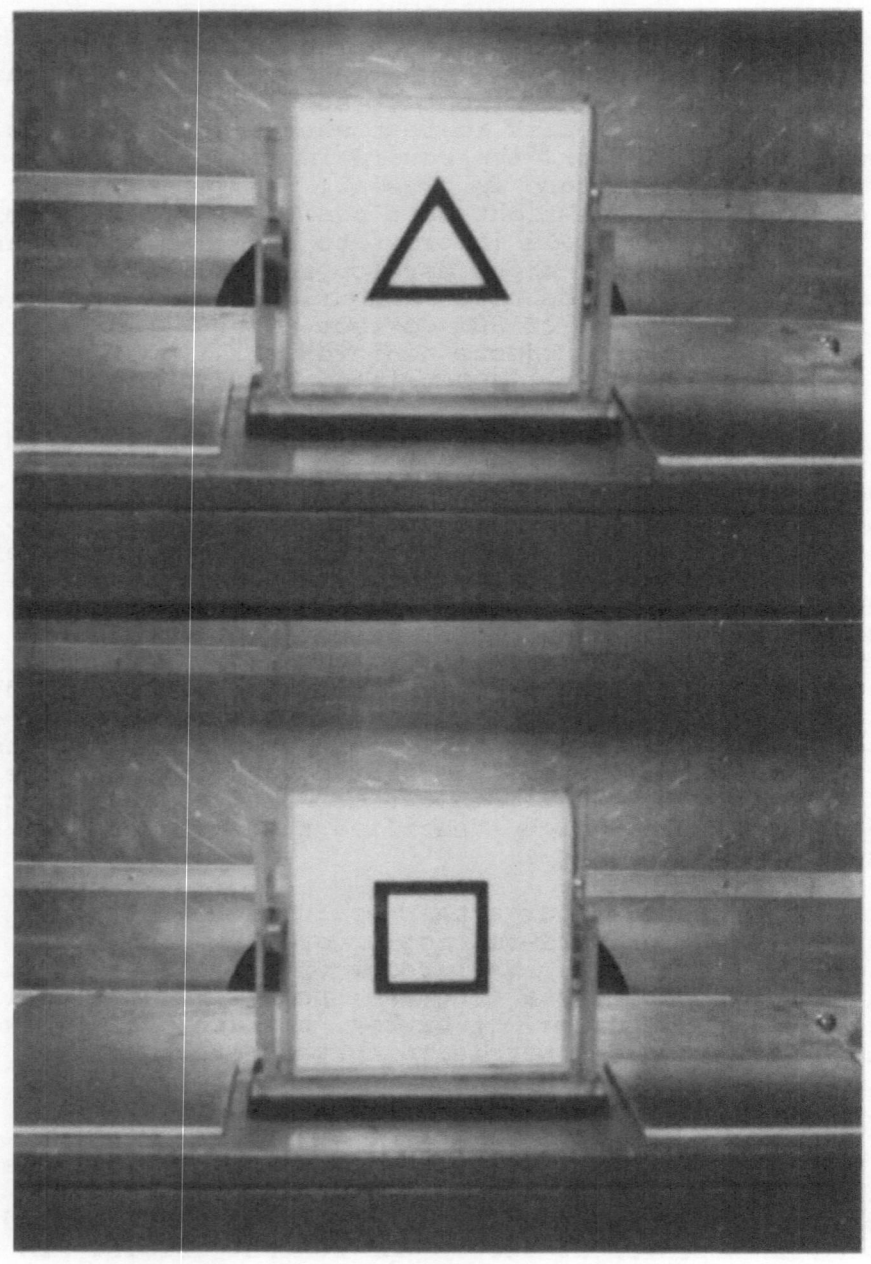

FIGURE 14. Stimuli used in conditional discrimination problem. Reward was under gray plaques to the left or right of the stimulus.

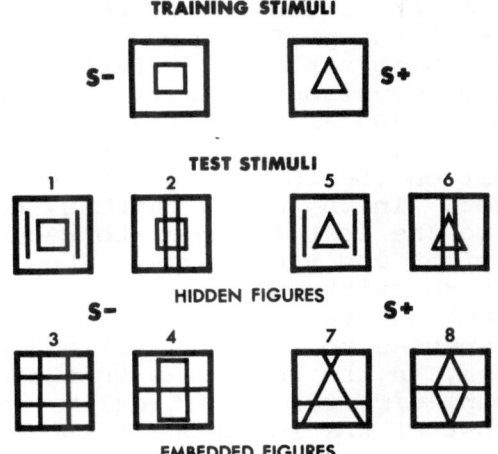

FIGURE 15. Training stimuli and transfer stimuli used
in the discrimination of embedded and hidden
figures

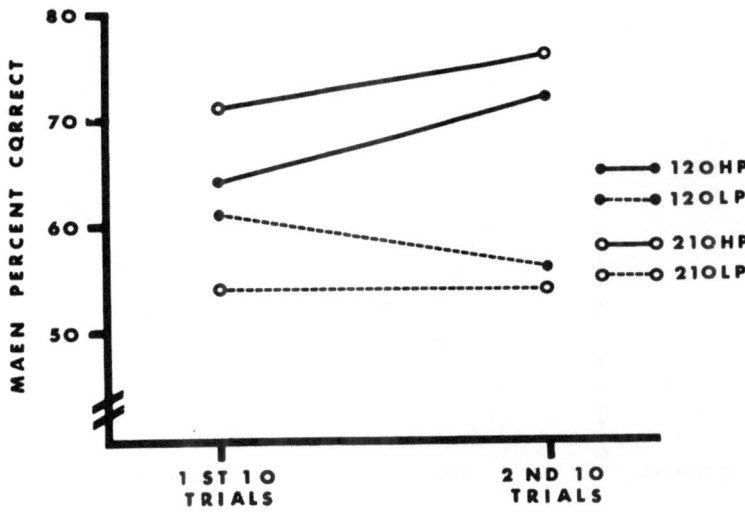

FIGURE 16. Mean percent of correct responses of the 120-
low- and high-protein-reared and 210-low- and
high-protein-reared monkeys on transfer to
embedded and hidden figures in the first ten
and last ten trials of testing.

The results of the attentional experiments led to the speculation that the performance on a pattern-strings task would also serve to differentiate the control from the malnourished monkeys. The pattern-string problems employed are illustrated in Figure 17. In the parallel and pseudocross problem, the animal merely has to pull on the chain nearest the reinforcement to be correct. In the cross pattern, however, the subject must go to the left in order to secure a reward which is on the right and <u>vice versa</u>. Thus, in the cross pattern, there exists a spatial discontiguity between reinforcement and response. The groups did not differ in the responses to the parallel and pseudocross problems. However, in the responses to the cross pattern, the groups differed dramatically--as can be seen in Figure 18. Most of the low-protein subjects responded significantly below chance in the early phases of testing on the cross pattern and finally adopted a position preference, settling for 50% reinforcement.

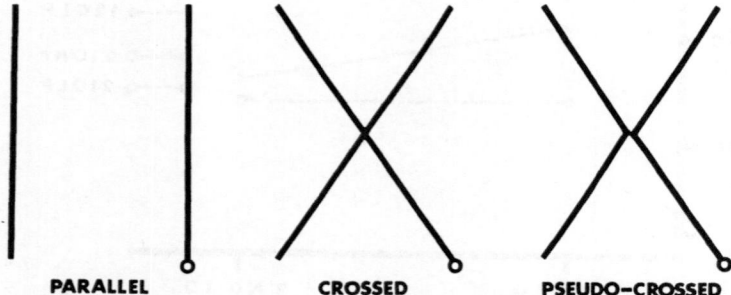

PARALLEL   CROSSED   PSEUDO-CROSSED

FIGURE 17. Pattern-strings problems.

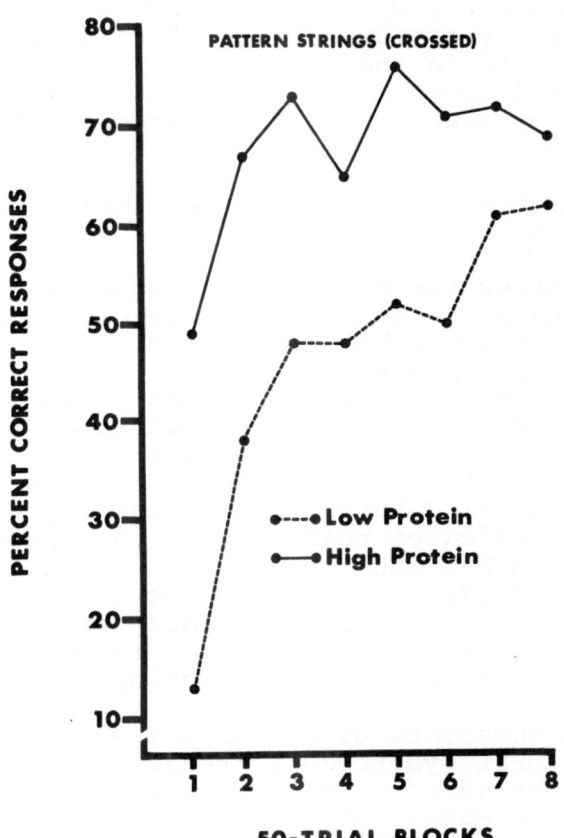

FIGURE 18. Percent correct responses of high- and
low-protein monkeys on the cross-strings
problems (over 400 trials). Note how
the low-protein-reared monkeys begin the
problem far below chance.

The results of the studies discussed above may be summarized as follows. The dietary variable does not appear to affect the performance of the developing malnourished monkey on delay response, learning set, long- or short-term memory, object discrimination, object-quality discrimination, or simple reversal learning. However, the dietary factor appears to be a highly significant variable in the responses of the low-protein animals to new and novel sources of stimulation and in all tasks which produce a stimulus-response, stimulus-reinforcement, or response-reinforcement discontiguity, such as reversal learning to central-cue stimuli, conditional learning, embedded-figures task, and cross-string problems.

With respect to the neural correlates of behavior, some speculation may be generated concerning potential organic loci for these behavioral deficiencies. The performance of delay response and the failure to find hyperactivity in the low-protein subjects would tend to support the contention that the frontal lobes are functioning adequately. Normal performance on memory tests suggest that the temporal lobes have not been affected. The normal development of learning sets and oddity learning indicates that perhaps the prestriate area of the cortex has not been affected. The adequate performance on the parallel and pseudocross-pattern strings task suggests normal functioning of the occipital area. In short, there is no indication that any neocortical areas are not functioning adequately.

The neural substrate of the protein-calorie malnutrition behavioral syndrome is probably located in the paleocortex or subcortical structures. The neophobic response--emotional responsiveness to strange stimuli--and the hyperreactivity to aversive stimulation is typical of an organism that has impaired amygdala function or an involvement of some aspect of the limbic system. The series of studies demonstrating impaired performance on tasks requiring attention or failure to cope with stimulus-response discontiguity direct attention to the possible abnormal functioning of hypocampal structures. One of the characteristics of animals with hypocampal lesions is a proneness to demonstrate disinhibition when a strange stimulus is introduced into a conditioning task. Low-protein animals which were trained on a two-minute fixed interval schedule for positive reinforcement until the rate of response during

the first minute of the time period was very low,
responded with great vigor when an auditory stimulus
was introduced in the first-minute segment of the time
interval. To the contrary, high-protein monkeys showed
a suppression of response (Strobel, 1972). These are,
of course, rather extreme speculations. Nevertheless,
the present research demonstrates that behavioral
deficiencies which can impair cognitive performance in
the developing rhesus monkey do appear as a result of
protein-calorie malnutrition.

A final speculation concerns a projection of the
present results to the human model. It is quite
evident that a child who finds new things in the
environment aversive, has deficiencies in curiosity and
manipulation and cannot deal with stimulus-response
discontiguities in an efficient manner would be at a
serious disadvantage in the modern world. Learning
which requires an organism to be attentive and flexible
would be impaired, and the child would be unable to
develop his full cognitive, intellectual, and social
potential.

ACKNOWLEDGMENTS

We would like to express our appreciation to
Raymond Guest, Edward Shea and Wanda Gordon whose
tireless efforts made this research possible. Research and preparation of this manuscript was supported in part by a grant from the Nutrition Foundation
Inc., #401, and Grant No. HD-04863 from the National
Institute of Child Health and Human Development.

REFERENCES

Aakre, B., Strobel, D. A., Zimmermann, R. R., and
    Geist, C. R., 1973, "Reactions to intrinsic and
    extrinsic rewards in protein-malnourished monkeys,"
    Percept. Mot. Skills 36:787-790.
Barnes, R. H., 1972, "Experimental studies in animals:
    Physiological and behavioral correlates of mal-
    nutrition," in: Nutrition, Growth, and Development
    of North American Indian Children (W. M. Moore,
    M. M. Silverberg, and M. S. Reid, eds.), pp. 121-128,
    Department of Health, Education and Welfare Pub-
    lication No. (NIH) 72-26, Washington, D. C.

Barnes, R. H., Cunnold, S. R., Zimmermann, R. R.,
    Simmons, H., MacLeod, R. B., and Krook, L., 1966,
    "Influences of nutritional deprivations in early
    life on learning behavior of rats as measured by
    performance in a water maze," J. Nutr. 89:399-410.
Behar, M., 1968, "Prevalence of malnutrition among
    preschool children of developing countries," in:
    Malnutrition, Learning, and Behavior (N. S. Scrimshaw
    and J. E. Gordon, pp. 30-41, Massachusetts Institute
    of Technology Press, Cambridge, Massachusetts.
Brockman, L. M., and Ricciuti, H. N., 1971, "Severe
    protein-calorie malnutrition and cognitive develop-
    ment in infancy and early childhood," Dev. Psychol.
    4:312-319.
Coursin, D. B., 1965, "Effect of undernutrition on CNS
    function," Nutr. Rev. 23:65.
Cravioto, J., 1968, "Nutritional deficiencies and
    mental performance in childhood," in: Environmental
    Influences (D. C. Glass, ed.), pp. 3-51, Rockefeller
    University Press, New York.
Cravioto, J., and Robles, B., 1963, "The influence of
    protein-calorie malnutrition on psychological test
    behavior," in: Mild-Moderate Forms of Protein-Calorie
    Malnutrition (G. Blix, ed.), pp. 115-125, Amqvist
    and Wiksells, Uppsala, Sweden.
Cravioto, J., and Robles, B., 1965, "Evolution of
    adaptive and motor behavior during rehabilitation
    from kwashiorkor," Am. J. Orthopsychiatry
    35:449-464.
Fantz, R. L., 1965, "Ontogeny of perception," in:
    Behavior of Nonhuman Primates, Volume 2 (A. M.
    Schrier, H. F. Harlow, and R. Stollnitz, eds.),
    pp. 365-404, Academic Press, New York.
Geist, C. R. Zimmermann, R. R., and Strobel, D. A.,
    1972, "Effect of protein-calorie malnutrition on
    food consumption, weight gain, serum proteins, and
    activity in the developing rhesus monkey (Macaca
    mulatta)," Lab. Anim. Sci. 22:369-377.
Harlow, H. F., and Harlow, M. K., 1965, "The affectional
    systems," in: Behavior of Nonhuman Primates, Volume 2
    (A. M. Schrier, H. F. Harlow, and F. Stollnitz eds.),
    pp. 405-448, Academic Press, New York.
Klein, R. E., Gilbert, O., Canosa, C., and DeLeon, R.,
    1969, "Performance of malnourished children in com-
    parison with adequately nourished children," Paper
    presented at the Annual Meeting of the American
    Association for the Advancement of Science.

Levitsky, D. A., and Barnes, R. H., 1972, "Nutritional and environmental interactions in the early development of the rat: Long-term behavioral effects," Science 176:68-71.

Monckeberg, F., 1968, "Effect of early marasmic malnutrition on subsequent physical and psychological development," in: Malnutrition, Learning, and Behavior (N. S. Scrimshaw and J. E. Gordon, eds.), pp. 269-278, M. I. T. Press, Cambridge, Massachusetts.

Peregoy, P. L., Zimmermann, R. R., and Strobel, D. A., 1972, "Protein preference in protein-malnourished monkeys," Percept. Mot. Skills 35:494-503.

Pollitt, E., 1972, "Behavioral correlates of severe malnutrition in man," in: Nutrition, Growth, and Development of North American Indian Children (W. M. Moore, M. M. Silverberg, and M. S. Reid, eds.), pp. 151-166, Department of Health, Education, and Welfare Publication No. (NIH) 76-26, Washington, D. C.

Rumbaugh, D. M., and Pournelle, M. E., 1966, "Discrimination-reversal skills of primates: The reversal-acquisition ratio as a function of phyletic standing," Psychonomic Sci. 1966, 4:45-46.

Stoch, M. B., and Smythe, P. J., 1963, "Does undernutrition during infancy inhibit brain growth and subsequent intellectual development?" Arch. Dis. Child. 38:546.

Stoch, M. B., and Smythe, P. J., 1968, "Undernutrition during infancy, and subsequent brain growth and development," in: Malnutrition, Learning, and Behavior (N. S. Scrimshaw and J. E. Gordon, eds.), pp. 278-288, M.I.T. Press, Cambridge, Massachusetts.

Stoffer, G., and Zimmermann, R. R., 1973, "Development of avoidance learning sets in normal and malnourished monkeys," Behav. Biol. 9:695-705.

Strobel, D. A., 1972, "Stimulus change and attentional variables as factors in the behavioral deficiency of malnourished, developing monkeys (Macaca mulatta)," Unpublished doctoral dissertation, University of Montana, Missoula, Montana.

Strobel, D. A., and Zimmermann, R. R., 1972, "Responsiveness of protein-deficient monkeys to manipulative stimuli," Devel. Psychobiol. 5:291-296.

Wells, A. M., Geist, C. R., and Zimmermann, R. R., 1972, "The influence of environmental and nutritional factors on problem solving in the rat," Percept. Mot. Skills 35:235-244.

Wise, L. A., and Zimmermann, R. R., 1973, "Shock thresholds of low- and high-protein reared rhesus monkeys," Percept. Mot. Skills 36:674.

Zimmermann, R. R., 1969a, "Early weaning and weight gain in infant rhesus monkeys," Lab. Anim. Care 19:644-647.

Zimmermann, R. R., 1969b, "Effects of age, experience and malnourishment on object retention in learning set," Percept. Mot. Skills 28:867-876.

Zimmermann, R. R., 1973, "Reversal learning in the developing, malnourished rhesus monkey," Behav. Biol. 8:281-390.

Zimmermann, R. R., and Geist, C. R., 1973, "A highly palatable and easy to make diet for producing protein-calorie malnutrition in the rhesus monkey," Laboratory Primate Newsletter 11:1-3.

Zimmermann, R. R., and Strobel, D. A., 1969, "Effects of protein-calorie malnutrition on visual curiosity, manipulation and social behavior in the infant rhesus monkey," Proceedings of the 77th Annual Convention of the American Psychological Association, pp. 241-242.

Zimmermann, R. R., Strobel, D. A., and Maguire, D., 1970, "Neophobic reactions in protein-malnourished infant monkeys," Proceedings of the 78th Annual Convention of the American Psychological Association, pp. 187-188.

Zimmermann, R. R., and Torrey, C. C., 1965, "Ontogeny of learning," in: Behavior of Nonhuman Primates, Volume 2 (A. M. Schrier, H. F. Harlow, F. Stollnitz eds.), pp. 405-448, Academic Press, New York.

Zimmermann, R. R., and Wells, A. M., 1971, "Performance of malnourished rats on the Hebb-Williams closed-field maze learning task," Percept. Mot. Skills, 33:1043-1050.

NUTRITION AND BRAIN DEVELOPMENT

Myron Winick

Director, Institute of Human Nutrition
Columbia University College of Physicians
and Surgeons
New York, N.Y.

It has long been known that malnutrition retards
growth. However, when these observations were initially
made, it was not clear whether or not a child would recover if he or she subsequently received adequate
nourishment. In an experiment done in Cambridge by
Kennedy, McCance, and Widdowson, two groups of rats were
malnourished for a period of time during growth. The
only difference between the two groups was that in one
the malnutrition was imposed from birth to weaning, and
in the second malnutrition was imposed later, during
the growth period. The results demonstrated that the
animals malnourished from birth until weaning were small
at the end of the period of malnutrition and remained
small throughout the rest of their lives, no matter how
they were subsequently fed. However, the group malnourished later in the growing period although also small
at the end of the period of malnutrition, caught up when
refed. So these investigators introduced the element of
time into the equation: the earlier the malnutrition, the
greater the chance of permanent effect. And yet, when
growth was examined in terms of weight or height, or the
usual anthropomorphic measurements, we could not break
it down in such a way as to explain this dichotomy in
recovery.

In 1962, Enesco and LeBlond were studying growth in
another way. They were simply asking the question: when
any organ grows, is it growing because it is increasing

65

in its number of component parts (number of cells), or
is it growing because the size of the already existing
components (the size of the cells) is increasing? Since
the DNA content of every diploid cell in a particular
species is a constant, and since that constant is known,
then simply by analyzing a total organ for DNA and dividing by the DNA content per cell, the number of cells
at any time in any organ could be calculated. Then by
weighing the organ, or doing a total protein content on
the organ, and dividing by the number of cells, a figure
for weight per cell, or the protein content per cell
(which is a rough measure of the size of the cell) could
be calculated. To restate this, DNA is located mainly
in the nucleus; it is constant in the diploid cell of
all species; and whether we divide by the constant or
not, it reflects cell number. Further, the protein or
weight/DNA ratio would reflect the weight or protein
per cell or cell size. The RNA/DNA ratio, for example,
would reflect the quantity of RNA per cell and anything
that is intracellular, when related to the DNA content,
would reflect the amount of that material per cell.

How then does the normal rat grow in these terms?
Growth in terms of organ size or weight stops at about
100 days postnatally, or 120 days after conception. But
the number of cells reaches a maximum before growth stops
in all the organs. The time in which this occurs varies
from organ to organ. In the brain, this occurs very
early, around 21 days postnatally. But in all the organs,
before growth stops, there is a period of time in which
the size of the organ is increasing, but the number of
cells is not. Therefore, the size of the individual cell
is increasing. If we look at growth carefully in these
terms, we can see three phases of growth. In the first
phase, total DNA content is increasing (cell division is
occurring) and total protein content is increasing at
the same rate. Therefore, the ratio is not changing,
cell size is not changing, and hyperplasia is occurring
alone. In the next phase, there is a reduction of the
rate of DNA synthesis and no change in the rate of net
protein synthesis. Therefore the ratio begins to increase, and hyperplasia and hypertrophy occur together.
During the last phase, DNA synthesis stops and net protein synthesis still continues. Hypertrophy occurs
alone.

One can now ask the question, do these three phases
of growth represent a possible explanation for the
"catch-up" phenomenon which we talked about? To test

this, we simply repeated the experiments of McCance and
Widdowson. We took three groups of animals and malnourished them for the same period of time, 21 days; the
only difference was the point at which we imposed the
malnutrition. In the first group, malnutrition was imposed from birth to 21 days, when all of the organs are
growing by hyperplasia; in the second group, malnutrition
was imposed from 22-43 days postnatally, when all the
organs are growing by hyperplasia except the brain and
lung; and in the third group, from 65-86 days, when all
of the organs are growing by cell enlargement. We then
examined these organs at the end of the period of malnutrition and after we had rehabilitated the animals.
At the end of the period of malnutrition in the first
group, a roughly proportional reduction in weight,
protein, RNA, and DNA was found. DNA was down, the
number of cells was down, and the ratios were relatively
normal. We had not affected the size of the cell. If
we refed these animals, they remained with a deficit in
number of cells. In the second group, again there was
a deficit in the number of cells in all of the organs,
except the brain and the lung. They reached their
normal number of cells before we began the experiment.
In these organs, the ratio or the size of the cell was
reduced, and if we refed these animals, the brain and
the lung recovered. The rest of the organs were left
with a deficit in the number of cells. In the last group,
in every case, the number of cells was normal before we
started the experiment, and it was the size of the cell
which was reduced. Refeeding these animals resulted in
recovery of all of the organs. So for this system, the
rat, we can say that malnutrition imposed during the
period of cell division will retard the rate of cell
division, and these changes will be permanent. However,
malnutrition during the period of cell enlargement will
prevent that enlargement, and if the animal is refed,
the cells will refill with protein and resume their normal
size.

These data suggest a general principle. Here is an
environmental stimulus which is, in fact, at least par-
tially determining the number of cells that any organ will
have. One can actually manipulate the rate of cell division simply by manipulating the nutrition during the
period of time that cells are dividing. For example, one
can superfeed animals from birth until weaning (another
technique perfected by McCance and Widdowson), and the
"superfed" or experimental animals have an increased
number of cells at the end of the period of superfeeding.

So it is possible to manipulate the rate of cell division
in either direction, within limits, of course, based on
the nutrition of the animal during the period of time the
cells are actually dividing.

This raises many questions. If we are interested
in the brain, we must remember that the brain is not a
homogeneous organ--it is made up of different cell types
and different regions. One can ask, are these principles
true for all regions of the brain and for all cell types?
In the rat the most rapid rate of cell division is in the
cerebellum, and it stops at about 17 days postnatal.
Cell division in the cerebrum is slower and will level
off at about 21 days. The brain stem shows very little
increase after 14 days, and there is a discrete increase
in the hippocampus which occurs between the 14th and the
17th day. This increase is not due to cell division in
the hippocampus, but to a migration of cells from under
the lateral ventricle into the hippocampus which has been
shown to occur on the 15th day of life. Thus, if we are
going to concern ourselves with the effects of malnutrition on cellular growth of the brain, we must concern
ourselves not only with cell division, but with cell
migration.

What happens if we malnourish an animal from birth?
The cerebellum is affected first and most seriously. The
cerebrum is affected later and not to the same degree,
and the migration of cells from under the lateral ventricle into the hippocampus is perhaps prevented. These
and a whole host of later studies demonstrate a general
principle: it does not make any difference what the
region of study is, what is important is the rate of
cell division in that region at the time that the stimulus is imposed. In this case, the cerebellum has the
most rapid rate of cell division and is affected the
most. What about the cell types involved? Using radio-
autography we can identify the cell types involved.
Malnutrition imposed at birth does not affect neuronal
division in the cerebral cortex, because neurons do not
divide postnatally. In the cerebellum, all three cell
types are affected and the primitive cells under the
lateral ventricle and under the third ventricle are
affected. These are the cells which migrate to the
hippocampus. Again, this demonstrates a general principle: it does not make any difference what the cell type
is, what is important is whether or not that cell type is
dividing when undernutrition is imposed. In effect then,
we are dealing with a fundamental stimulus to cell division.

Let us examine some of the possible mechanisms involved in this process. It is possible that one reason
why DNA synthesis is reduced is because the enzymatic
machinery necessary for the synthesis of DNA is impaired.
DNA polymerase is theoretically involved in the terminal
phase of the synthesis of the DNA molecule. Whether or
not its activity increases as a consequence of DNA
synthesis, or whether increased activity causes DNA
synthesis is controversial. There are some data which
shed light on this controversy. During normal growth,
activity of the enzyme correlates with the rate of cell
division in the brain, so that this enzyme is a good
marker for the rate of cell division. If we look at the
various regions of the brain, again we see this parallel.
In the cerebellum, where there are two peaks of cell
division, one believed to be neuronal, and the other
believed to be glial, two peaks in the activity of DNA
polymerase are observed. So again the enzyme reflects
the rate of cell division. If an animal is malnourished,
the activity of this enzyme is reduced. So far, the
enzyme mirrors the rate of cell division, and malnutrition lowers the activity of the enzyme. If we attempt
to rehabilitate an animal during the period when cells
can still rapidly divide, the animal will tend to show
catchup growth for awhile, by accelerating the rate of
cell division. By this mechanism the organs begin to
make up the deficit in the reduced number of cells. It
takes two days of refeeding under these experimental
conditions before an increased rate of DNA synthesis or
cell division is seen. But if we measure the activity
of DNA polymerase, there is a very marked increase above
the normal activity within 24 hr of refeeding. This has
clearly occurred before any changes in DNA synthesis is
measured either by incorporation of C^{14} thymidine or by
total DNA analysis. At 48 hr, DNA synthesis increases
and enzyme activity remains high. Therefore, the activity of this enzyme increases prior to any increase in
cell division. We are therefore suggesting that malnutrition interferes selectively with the synthesis of
this particular protein and that an effect of this reduced enzymatic activity is a retarded rate of cell
division.

Another mechanism which could retard DNA synthesis
is reduced availability of nucleotides. Examining that
possibility reveals that the total nucleotide-pool size
increases during development, but that malnutrition has
no effect on the nucleotide-pool size in the brain. We
therefore can not say that the reduced amount of RNA or

DNA is due to fewer total nucleotides. However, if we examine the incorporation of amino acids into the brain-nucleotide pool, we find, surprisingly, that the malnourished animal incorporates amino acids at a faster rate. So in order to keep that pool size constant, amino acids enter more rapidly and nucleotides exit from the pool more rapidly into RNA; RNA synthesis is actually increased. By contrast, nucleotides enter into DNA more slowly. Thus, the "availability" of nucleotides for DNA synthesis decreases a second mechanism in the reduction of cell division. We have an increase in RNA synthesis with RNA content dropping. RNA catabolism increases more than the increased synthesis. The level of RNA, therefore, seems to be controlled by the catabolic phase. For this reason, one might study the enzymes involved in RNA catabolism, for example, alkaline RNase. Activity of this enzyme is markedly elevated in the brains of malnourished rats.

At this point it can be said that malnutrition affects protein synthesis not only generally, but by altering the activity of specific enzymes involved in RNA metabolism and in the synthesis of DNA.

One issue that always confronts those of us who work with experimental animals is the relevance of our experiments to the situation in the human. Normal cellular growth has been studied in the human brain. Data were collected in New York City from children who died of accidents, poisonings, crib deaths, and some therapeutic abortions; in other words, normal children who died of some catastrophic event. These data showed that brain weight and protein and RNA content increases in early infancy until at least one year of age, by contrast, DNA content increases before birth, then begins to level off, and by almost one year of age, all the cells necessary have been laid down. Thus, if we are concerned with the effects of malnutrition on cellular growth of the brain, we must concern ourselves with that form of malnutrition prevalent during the first year of life, i.e., the child with severe marasmus. If such a child dies, the weight or the protein content of the brain is reduced. In addition, the number of cells in the brain is also reduced when compared to children who died of accidents or crib deaths. Thus, early malnutrition in a human will retard cell division in the developing brain. We do not know whether or not these children could have recovered from this. But all of the experience in pigs, rats and dogs indicates that

this change is permanent, unless the rehabilitation
starts when cell division is still occurring. In the
human brain, DNA synthesis in the cerebrum is more
rapid than in the cerebellum postnatally. In the
cerebrum, cerebellum, and brain stem, cell division
stops at around 12-18 months postnatally. Malnutrition
in the human during the first 12-18 months reduces the
number of cells quite dramatically in all three of
these areas. Again, we see the fundamental principle--
that if cells are dividing, malnutrition will reduce
this rate.

In rat brain and human brain, myelin synthesis is
reduced by malnutrition. Both total cholesterol and
phospholipid content are reduced in human brain.
Moreover, if we relate the myelin to the number of
cells, we find early that there is no reduction in
myelin per cell. In other words, the reduction in the
rate of cell division and myelination are proportional.
The amount of myelin per cell remains relatively constant, but then, myelination continues longer than cell
division and if the malnutrition persists, the amount
of myelin per cell drops. These data are very similar
to the data we collected in pigs and rats. Certain
clinical measurements are easier to make in the human
than in animals. For example, head circumference can
be accurately measured. This has been very useful in
looking at the growth of the brain. Malnutrition will
result in marked reduction in head circumference. However, when the weight of the brain is plotted against
the head circumference, the malnourished and normal
children fall on the same curve. In other words, the
reduced head circumference reflects the weight of the
brain accurately, regardless of whether the child is
malnourished or not. In fact, head circumference
accurately reflects the total protein and total DNA
contents of the brain.

Let us now examine malnutrition occurring before
birth. Suppose we malnourish a rat for the entire
period of life when his brain cells are dividing: from
conception to 21 days postnatally. Prenatal malnutrition alone in the rat reduces the number of cells at
birth by about 15%; postnatal malnutrition alone in the
rat reduces the number of cells in the brain by about
15% at weaning. The combined effect of these two forms
of deprivation produce a reduction of 60% in the number
of cells. So that not only is the time of the malnutrition important, but the duration within that time span
is also critically important.

Now, what do we know about prenatal malnutrition in
the human? One tissue which has been studied is the
placenta, and in a rat it has been shown that the placenta exhibits changes with prenatal malnutrition similar
to the organs of the rat subjected to early postnatal
malnutrition. Data collected in Equador indicate that
in human placentae from malnourished women, the activity
of alkaline RNase (which is high in malnourished tissues)
is markedly elevated. Malnutrition has been shown to
reduce the number of cells in the placentae from malnourished women.

Does prenatal malnutrition affect the human fetal
brain? Here the evidence is indirect. If we look at
the number of cells in the brains of children who died
of severe malnutrition, and were subsequently studied,
we find two major groups: the child with marasmus who
is malnourished in the first year of life, and the
child with kwashiorkor who is, more often than not,
malnourished in the second or third year of life after
being taken off the breast. In a child with kwashiorkor,
the number of cells in the brain, as we might predict,
is normal. The size of the cell is reduced. In the
marasmic children, the number of cells is reduced.
However, the marasmic children can be divided into two
groups. In one group there is a 15% reduction, whereas
in the second group there is a 60% reduction. The
differences between these two groups is that in those
with a 15% reduction, the child was of normal birth
weight and then became malnourished; whereas in the
group with the 60% reduction, the child weighed less
than 2000 g (5 lb) at birth. It is conceivable that
this is a premature infant, and the premature infant is
more susceptible to malnutrition, or it is equally conceivable that this represents the clinical counterpart
of the double-deprived rat that was shown earlier, and
that this child was malnourished both before and after
birth, resulting in a 60% reduction in the number of
cells.

To summarize, at the present we can clearly say that
malnutrition in animals will interfere with the rate of
cell division when cells are dividing in the brain, in
all regions and in all cell types, and it will be accom-
plished by a mechanism involving a general and selective
effect on protein synthesis. Malnutrition prenatally in
the rat will result in precisely the same thing, and the
duration of the malnutrition will be more than additive,
at least in terms of the effects on the fetal brain.

Malnutrition in the human shortly after birth will reduce the rate of cell division and will result in a brain with fewer cells. In addition, myelination will also be curtailed. Malnutrition prenatally in the human will affect the rate of cell division in the placentae. Finally, there are some data which suggest that prenatal malnutrition in the human acts synergistically with postnatal malnutrition, curtailing cell division and therefore resulting in a brain with a marked reduction in cell number.

REFERENCES

Scrimshaw, N. S., and Gordon, J. E., eds., 1968, Malnutrition, **Learning**, and **Behavior, M.I.T. Press,** Cambridge, Mass.

Winick, M., 1969, "Malnutrition and brain development," J. Pediatr. 74:667-679.

Winick, M., 1970, "Nutrition and mental development," Med. Clin. North Am. 54:1413-1429.

Winick, M., ed., 1972, Current **Concepts in Nutrition,** Vol. 1, Nutrition and Development, John Wiley and Sons, New York.

MALNUTRITION AND ANIMAL MODELS OF COGNITIVE DEVELOPMENT

David A. Levitsky

Division of Nutritional Sciences
     and
Department of Psychology
Cornell University
Ithaca, N.Y.

I would like to begin by saying that the work presented here and probably at some other points throughout the conference is a result of a close **collaborative** effort. It is a truly multidisciplinary effort between myself as a psychologist, **or more appropriately, a be-havorist, my students, and Dr. Richard H. Barnes, a well-known nutritionist, who is one of the pioneers in the study of nutrition and behavior.**

One of the first questions with which we concerned ourselves was the selection of the most appropriate animal model for the study of malnutrition and human cognitive development and, more importantly, mental retardation. The implicit model of human mental retardation which has been promulgated for some time in animal psychology is the simple learning model. Any variable which affects the ability of an animal to make associations between stimuli (learning) affects cognitive development in a similar fashion. More **explicitly, any** variable which produces a decrement in learning is taken as analogous to decrements in cognitive development, i.e., mental retardation.

The much quoted early studies of Cowley and Griesel (1959, 1962, 1963, 1964, 1966) were based on this model. Their studies showed that rats malnourished from early life displayed deficits in simple learning ability. Besides the assumption that simple learning ability is

75

analogous to human cognitive development, they and many
others in the area at that time assumed that malnutrition produced a kind of brain damage and therefore a
breakdown in the "machinery of learning" (brain) such
that learning could not occur. Studies which demonstrated long term alteration in brain lipid and DNA
content were taken as confirmation of the breakdown in
the machinery of learning.

Testing the learning ability of animals is not
simple. Since we have no means to observe learning
directly, we are restricted to the observation of
learning vis-a-vis performance. However, there are
many variables which may affect performance and have
nothing to do with learning. One therefore must be
very careful not to draw false conclusions about the
effects of variables on learning from data acquired
through simple learning situations.

This problem is particularly serious in the study
of nutrition and learning, since we generally use nutrients as reinforcements for learning. We have observed
that malnutrition early in the life of the rat has a
long lasting effect on feeding and drinking behavior
(Levitsky and Barnes, 1969). If we do not use nutrient
reinforcement, then we generally use aversive stimulation
in learning situations. Unfortunately, we have observed
a difference in the reaction of malnourished rats to
aversive stimulation. Given almost any kind of aversive
stimulus, the previously malnourished rat exhibits an
exaggerated response to it (Levitsky and Barnes, 1970).
Because of these problems in differential effects of
either appetitive or aversive stimuli on the behavior of
the previously malnourished rats, it is extremely difficult to conclude from the literature that malnutrition has
any effect on simple learning ability in rats (Levitsky
and Barnes, 1973). We therefore set forth a program in
which we questioned whether there is any effect of early
malnutrition on learning ability when all possible performance variables are controlled.

Basically our nutritional design was to expose an
animal to very severe malnutrition early in life. As
soon as dams gave birth, we allowed them access only to
a 12% casein diet (10% protein) for the three weeks of
lactation. At birth the pups were randomly assigned to
each dam and reduced to 8 per litter. After 21 days of
lactation the pups were weaned and placed on a 3% casein
diet for the next four weeks. It should be reemphasized

that this was a very severe bout of malnutrition. There
was very little growth during this period of malnutrition.
We allowed recovery, and as Dr. Winick pointed out, recovery of body weight was never complete. We always
obtained a decrement of 18-20% in body weight. In order
to study the effects of early malnutrition we allowed at
least 10 weeks recovery, because we wanted to see whether
we could produce a permanent change in brain structure
and this learning mechanism.

We designed a learning situation (visual discrimination) in which we used food as a reinforcement, but we
also could assess and control the food motivation of our
animals. The apparatus, a modified Skinner box, is
schematically represented in Figure 1. We first deprived
the animals of food and placed them in the apparatus with
only the single center bar protruding into the testing cage.
The animals readily learned to press the bar to obtain a
45 mg food pellet. The reinforcement schedule was a
VI-1' which delivered a food pellet on the average of once
every minute if the animal pressed the center bar. All
animals readily learned this task. We used the rate of
bar pressing as an index of food motivation.

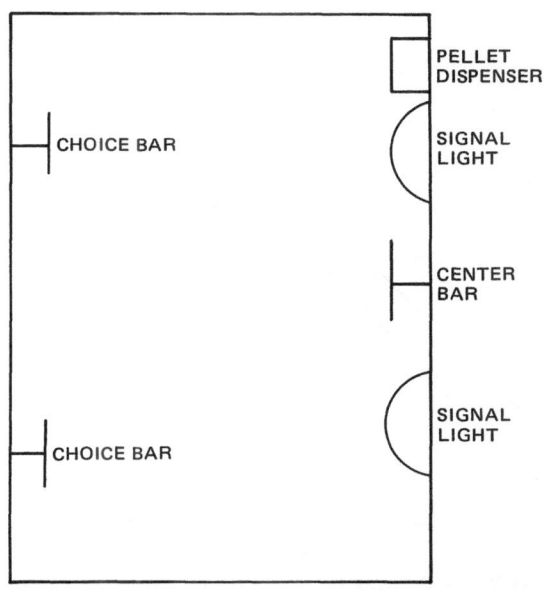

FIGURE 1. Diagram of testing chamber.

If one then plots the rate of bar pressing as a
function of the amount of weight loss, one obtains a
linear logarithmic function, but as can be seen
from Figure 2, the malnourished animals were much more
sensitive to the food deprivation, responding at a greater
rate for the same weight loss when compared to controls.
We then selected a rate of bar pressing (motivation) and
titrated the amount of food that the animal received
following the testing session such that all animals
eventually produced approximately the same rate of bar
pressing, i.e., the same rate of motivation to solve the
problem. It was only after this training and stabiliza-
tion of motivational state that the discrimination problem was introduced.

The problem was one of visual discrimination.
When the animals pressed the center bar, instead of being
rewarded with a food pellet, one of the two lights on the
opposite wall became illuminated and the animal had to
turn around and press one of the bars on the same side

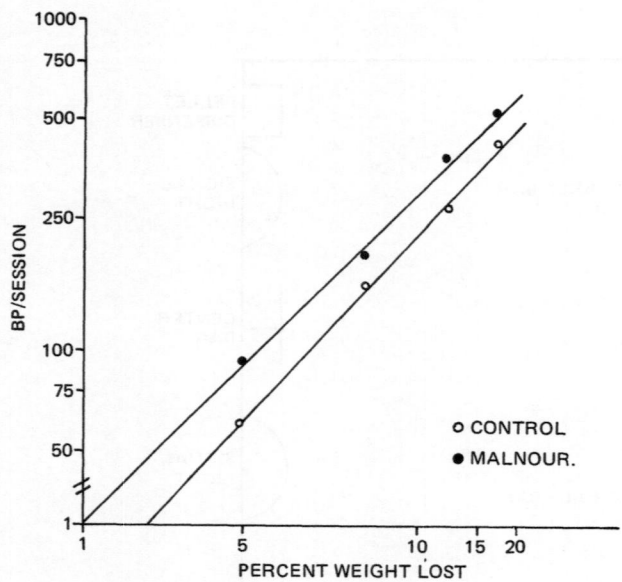

FIGURE 2. Mean total bar presses per session as a
          function of percent body weight loss for
          previously malnourished rats and controls.

as the illuminated light in order to obtain the food
pellet. The rat then could start a new trial by again
pressing the center bar. If the animal made an error,
it would again have to press the center bar to produce
a new trial (noncorrection method). We controlled for
the rate at which the animal presented the problem
by varying the amount of food the animal received
in his home cage following testing. We then analyzed
the number of correct responses per 50 trials through
the course of learning this visual discrimination problem. We observed no difference in learning rate in this
situation when we controlled for the rate of motivation.
We next arranged a reversal learning problem which has
been shown to be more sensitive, as Dr. Zimmermann mentioned, to various kinds of manipulation. The animals
now had to press the bar associated with the nonillumin-
ated light. Again, we observed no difference in the rate
at which the animals could learn the reversal problem.

We then considered the possibility that perhaps
short-term memory is affected by early malnutrition.
Using the same animals and apparatus, we exposed the
animals to an alternative problem, using the two back
bars. To solve the problem the animals had to press the
center bar and then turn around and depress one of the
back bars to obtain a food pellet. That ended the first
trial. To start the next trial the rat had to again
press the center bar, but in order to receive a food
pellet on this trial, the rat had to press the bar which
had not been pressed on the previous trial. Thus, in
order to respond correctly, the animal would have had to
recall its previous response. It should be pointed out
that the rate of motivation was still being held as constant as possible. Under these conditions, the rate of
learning this kind of alteration behavior was a bit slower
for the previously malnourished rats. For the last 400
trials there was a significant (p < 0.05) difference. We
then increased the minimum time interval between trials.
Whereas in the free-responding situation the mean intertrial interval was 7.5 sec, we placed a minimum of 15
sec between trials. This means the animal, in order to
make a correct response, would have had to recall its
previous response over a minimum interval of 15 sec.
Again we obtained significant differences (p < 0.01); the
previously malnourished rats displayed less efficient
behavior. We were quite elated at this, thinking we had
found evidence of short-term memory deficits, and thus
proof that there is a permanent breakdown in the machinery of the central nervous system.

However, when we examined the records very carefully, we found that if the malnourished animal made a mistake, then the latency to return to press the center bar again was significantly greater than in the well-nourished controls. Moreover, after making a correct response the latency to respond was shorter, and since the next trial would not start, the animal pressed the back bars. We interpreted this effect as showing that the previously malnourished rats were more affected emotionally by the learning problem than were the well-nourished controls. This interpretation was consistent with all of our other observations of increased reactivity to aversive stimuli in the previously malnourished animals. Thus, what we found in this situation, we believe, was simply another reflection of increased behavioral reactivity in a stressful situation rather than a true memory deficit. These tests are important, however, in demonstrating that although our procedures were sensitive enough to show that these previously malnourished animals were different from controls, we could find no difference in learning when the level of motivation was carefully controlled.

These data raise a number of questions concerning our model of cognitive development, the learning model. Is it possible that our animal model is wrong, that is, that the rate of learning simple problems may not be a good measure of human cognitive development? There are data from human studies which suggest that even mentally retarded children given a simple discrete learning problem do not show any differences in the rate of making associations. It is possible that the rate of making associations (simple learning) may not be a true measure of a deficit in cognitive development, and thus, it may not be the most appropriate model for the study of the effects of malnutrition on cognitive development. If we believe that malnutrition does produce effects on human cognitive development, then we must find another model to explain the interaction between nutrition and behavior.

From a review of the literature we became aware that other manipulations experienced very early in life can produce the same kind of effects on behavior as we have observed with early malnutrition. If the rat and other mammals are environmentally isolated early in life, they also show long term increases in "emotional reactivity" as adults. Moreover, various kinds of environment stimulation, like group housing or experimenter handling, occurring early in life produce animals which display a diminished response to aversive stimulation as adults.

This similarity between early environmental and nutritional effects on behavior raised the possibility of a common mechanism responsible for the behavioral effects produced by these two apparently disparate variables.

We then decided to compare and interact early nutritional **and environmental conditions. We used six groups** of rats in a two by three factorial design. We used the same kind of nutritional conditions as described previously. The animals were malnourished **for the first seven weeks of life, or** given a control diet. **Superimposed** on these two nutritional conditions were three environmental conditions. A control environment was defined by weighing the animals once a week, changing the bedding three times a week, filling food cups three or four times per week, and weaning the animal to individual cages. Our stimulated animals were picked up every day and handled for about three min for the three weeks of lactation. They were weaned to two animals per cage instead of isolated cages for the next four weeks. Also, during this time they were exposed for one hr a day to a large playground with many different kinds of toys and five other animals of the same group. For the isolated conditions the animals were reared in soundproof, lightproof chambers during the three weeks of lactation and for four weeks postweaning. After seven weeks of experimental intervention, all the animals were placed in the control environment and received the control diet for twelve weeks. We then looked at their behavior.

We found that many kinds of behaviors were altered by the experimental treatment (Levitsky and Barnes, 1972), as exemplified by locomotor activity (Figure 3). The effects of malnutrition on locomotor activity were exacerbated by the environmental isolation conditions. For this particular behavior the effects of malnutrition were completely obliterated in the stimulation conditions. Other kinds of behavior which we observed did not show this complete obliteration, but in almost all cases, we showed that the effects of malnutrition can be exacerbated by putting the animals in an isolated environment.

The results of this study suggested to us the following model to exemplify how nutrition may affect cognitive development. It is quite clear from the literature that young mammals must "learn" a significant amount of information from the environment. It appears that the more developed the cortex (association areas) the greater the importance of this early experimental period for the

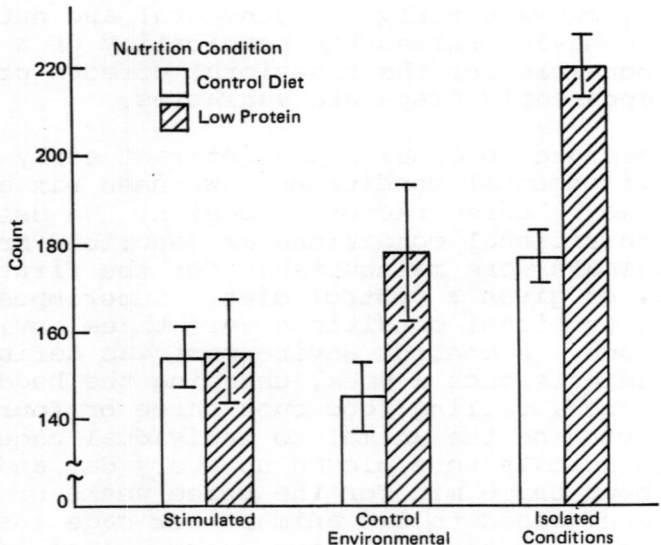

FIGURE 3. Mean and standard error of total locomotor movements per session for each treatment condition.

development of appropriate behavior as an adult. If the mammal is restricted from his environment during the important period of development, then adult behavior is severely altered. **The model which we suggest is that** malnutrition acts to produce its long term effects on behavior by "functionally isolating" the animal from his environment. From interaction studies it appears that it is possible to override this nutritionally-induced isolation with endogenous stimulation. But perhaps of greater significance is the fact that this diminution of endogenous environmental learning is exaggerated in environments containing a paucity of stimulation.

In order to test this model of nutritionally induced functional isolation, we examined the development of behavior during the period of malnutrition with particular attention being directed to the development of environmental exploratory behaviors. To do this, Mr. Thomas Massaro and I developed our "Automated Peeping-Tom" apparatus. The apparatus consisted of a 35 mm camera which was programmed to take a picture once every three minutes for a twelve-hour period. We then analyzed each frame and classified the behavior into various categories. The experimental technique turned out to be extremely sensitive primarily because there was no experimenter-subject interaction and we were able to collect a large number of observations per subject. Figure 4 shows the amount of time we observed the dam in the nesting area, expressed as a percentage of observation time. Unfortunately, we were unable to discriminate the pups suckling. We found that the control animals showed a gradual developmental decline in this response throughout the 28 days, whereas this decline was significantly decreased if the dam was maintained on a low-protein diet. We were expecting that maternal malnutrition would result in poorer mothers. Of course, we do not know if time spent with the young is a valid index of a good mother or not, but we have observed this effect repeatedly in our studies; malnourished dams spend much more time with their pups during the period of lactation.

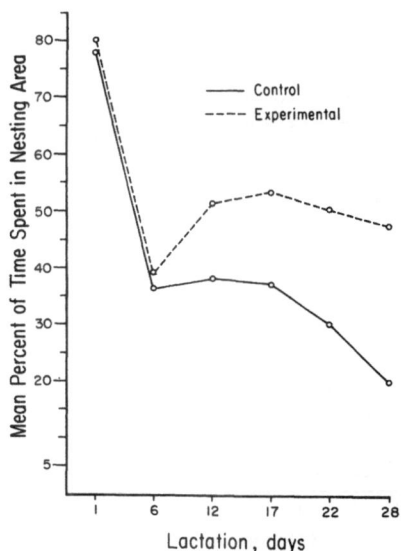

FIGURE 4. Mean percent of time spent in nesting area by dam over time as a function of nutritional treatment.

If one now looks at the development of the pups as
the lactation period progressed toward weaning, it is
clear that the pups spent less time in small groups.
Originally the pups were held in little packets of 8,
but as time proceeded we observed more of them separated.
The animals started exploring their environment. As can
be seen very clearly from Figure 5, malnourishing the
dam delayed the dispersal of the pups from the nesting
area. This observation supports in part our concept
that the mechanism through which malnutrition was affecting cognitive development in animals was by functionally
isolating the animal from his environment. The concept
is further supported by several reports showing a delayed
motor development of malnourished pups (Simonson **et al.**,
1969; Altman **et al**., 1970; Smart and Dobbing, 1971).
What we have shown here is the environmental consequence
both of the delayed motor development and the increased
maternal behavior of the dam.

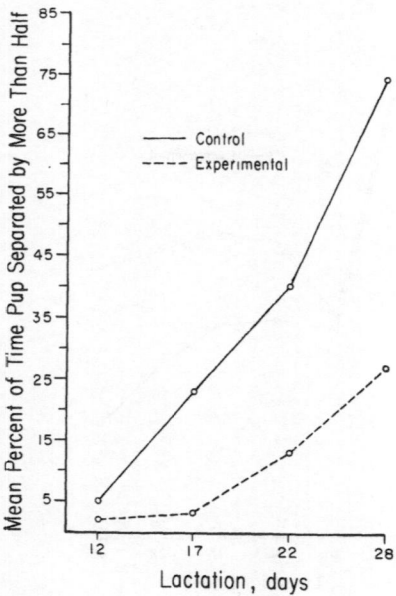

FIGURE 5. **Mean percent of observation in which the pups
             were observed in groups of 3 or less over the
             period of lactation.**

The development of feeding behavior is particularly interesting (Figure 6). This is defined as the percentage of time we observed the pups eating from the food cup. As with the development of other behaviors there is a depression in the development of this behavior. In this case, however, it is quite advantageous, since the ingestion of the low-protein diet would only present greater problems to the young developing animal.

Perhaps the best example of the inhibiting effect of **malnutrition on environmental exploration can be seen** in the severe retardation of climbing behavior (Figure 7). Before about day 22, very few observations of climbing behavior were made, but this behavior developed very rapidly after that **day in the controls. This developmental** rate, however, was dramatically depressed in the malnourished pups.

We have thus shown that malnutrition does produce decreases in the interaction between the young animal and his environment by delaying the onset of various kinds of behaviors which propel the animal from the maternal litter into the environment and by the increased maternal behavior which further acts in preventing the pups from exploring the environment. There exists another mechanism through which malnutrition also may act to isolate the young animal from its environment. Dr. Zimmermann has shown, as has Dr. Elias at Harvard, that a malnourished monkey **avoids, or at least does not** approach, **novel objects in his environment. We have also** observed this same phenomenon in both rats and pigs. This mechanism operates not only in the **preweaning animal,** but in the weaned animal as well. We are currently investigating this mechanism in further depth.

We have also observed another mechanism which may lead to **nutritionally-induced functional** isolation. We spoke earlier of endogenous learning, that is, the animal was not "required" to learn the information because of some reinforcement contingency. In previous learning studies discussed above, the animal was always required to learn the environmental information we presented in order to solve the problem. Early environmental learning, on the other hand, is not "demanded" but is endogenously stimulated. Psychologists have studied this problem under the labels of "latent learning" or "incidental learning." We then attempted to find out if malnutrition may also disrupt this process.

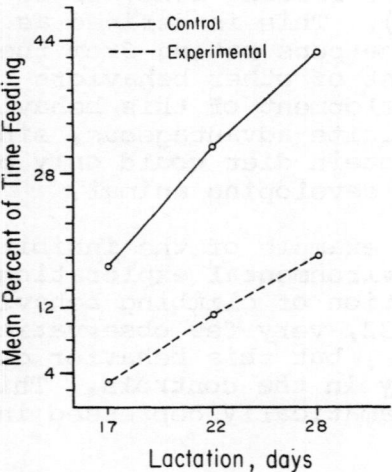

FIGURE 6. Mean percent of observations of pups feeding from food cup.

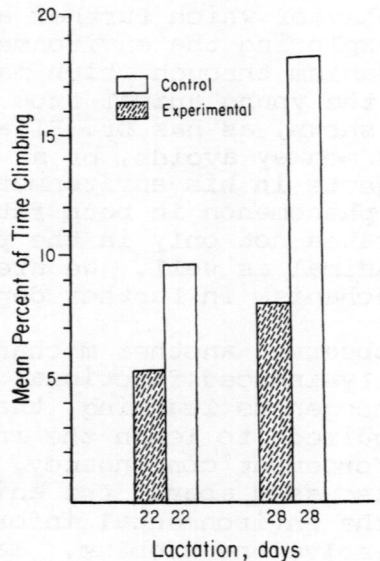

FIGURE 7. Mean percent of observations of pups climbing the sides of cage.

The procedure we followed was the classic procedure for demonstrating latent learning in rats. We first exposed young (4-week-old) rats to a maze. There were no reinforcements in the maze, i.e., food, water, etc. We allowed the animals to explore the maze in the first study for 7 hours and in a second study for 4 hours. We later made the animals hungry, put food at the end of the maze, and simply counted the number of errors committed by the animal in learning this maze for food. If the scores of these animals are compared to ones which did not have an opportunity to explore the maze (but were handled similarly), then the difference in errors may be attributed to the information gathered and utilized by the experienced animal in the learning situation. It is typically found that allowing a rat access to the maze substantially reduces the number of errors in learning the maze for a reinforcement.

We then asked, what happens if the animals are malnourished at the time they experience this maze? Table I represents the percent savings in learning the maze due to experience for both control and malnourished rats.

TABLE I. Percent Savings of Errors Due to Prior Maze Experience

	Experiment I	Experiment II
Control	69.3	46.0
Malnourished	45.0	21.3

It should be pointed out that during the time of experiencing the maze the animals had been maintained on a 7% casein diet. All animals had normal prenatal and postnatal nutrition. Furthermore, the animals were rehabilitated before testing. The control animals displayed a significantly greater savings in both experiments than the animals which were malnourished at the time of the original exposure to the maze. In most cases the animals which were malnourished but received experience in the maze did as poorly as the well nourished

animals with no experience in the maze. So for some
reason, the effect of experience in this maze was blocked
by malnutrition.

In summary, we believe that we have been using the
wrong animal model for the study of malnutrition and
human cognitive development. We previously assumed the
brain was permanently damaged as a result of early malnutrition and that this could be reflected by the rate
of learning a problem. We could find no evidence of a
detrimental effect of early malnutrition on rate of
learning when we carefully controlled for motivational
variables.

Currently, we feel that a programming model of
cognitive development may be a more suitable analogue.
Specifically, we suggested and offered some evidence in
support of this model by demonstrating at least three
mechanisms through which malnutrition may effectively
restrict the mammal from accumulating environmental
information early in life. Thus, the problem of
defining the mechanism through which nutrition affects
the brain and behavior should concentrate not on the
"ability" to learn, but on the "willingness" to learn,
particularly during the early part of life.

ACKNOWLEDGMENTS

This work has been supported in part by funds sup-
plied through the State University of New York by research
grant HD-02581 and Career Development Award HD-70510 from
the National Institute of Child Health and Human Development and the Nutrition Foundation.

REFERENCES

Altman, J., Sudarshan, K., Das, G. D., McCormick, N.,
   and Barnes, D., 1970, "The influence of nutrition on
   neural and behavioral development: III. Development
   of some motor, particularly locomotor patterns during
   infancy," Dev. Psychobiol. 4(2): 97-114.
Cowley, J. J., and Griesel, R. D., 1959, "Some effects
   of a low protein diet on a first filial generation
   of white rats," J. Genet. Psychol. 95: 187-201.
Cowley, J. J., and Griesel, R. D., 1962, "Pre- and postnatal effects of a low protein diet on the behavior of
   the white rat," Psychologia Af. 9: 216-225.

Cowley, J. J., and Griesel, R. D., 1963, "The develop-
ment of a second generation of low-protein rats,"
J. Genet. Psychol. 103: 233-242.
Cowley, J. J., and Griesel, R. D., 1964, "Low-protein
diet and emotionality in the albino rat," J. Genet.
Psychol. 104: 89-98.
Cowley, J. J., and Griesel, R. D., 1966, "The effect on
growth and behavior of rehabilitating first and
second generation low-protein rats," Anim. Behav. 14:
506-517.
Levitsky, D. A., and Barnes, R. H., 1969, "Effects of
early malnutrition on animal behavior," Am. Assoc.
Adv. Sci. Pub.
Levitsky, D. A., and Barnes, R. H., 1970, "Effects of
early malnutrition on the reaction of adult rats in
aversive stimulation," Nature 225: 468-469.
Levitsky, D. A., and Barnes, R. H., 1972, "Nutritional
and environmental interactions in the behavioral
development of the rat: long-term effects," Science
176: 68-71.
Levitsky, D. A., and Barnes, R. H., 1973, "Malnutrition
and animal behavior," in: Nutrition, Development and
Social Behavior, David J. Kallen (ed.), DHEW Pub.
No. (NIH) 73-242.
Simonson, M., Sherwin, R. W., Anilane, J. K., Yu, W. Y.,
and Chow, B. F., 1968, "Neuromotor development in
progeny of underfed mother rats," J. Nutr. 98:18-24.
Smart, J. L., and Dobbing, J., 1971, "Vulnerability of
developing brain. VI. Relative effects of foetal
and early postnatal undernutrition on reflex ontogeny
and development of behavior in the rat," Brain Res.
33: 303-314.

INTERACTIVE EFFECTS OF VARIABLE POPULATION DENSITY AND
DIETARY PROTEIN SUFFICIENCY UPON SELECTED MORPHOLOGICAL,
NEUROCHEMICAL, AND BEHAVIORAL ATTRIBUTES IN THE RAT

Robert W. Bell

Chairman, Department of Psychology
Texas Tech University
Lubbock, Texas

ABSTRACT

Rats were reared from weaning until 48 days of age
ranging from 2 to 30 animals per group. Multiples of
each group size were created and factorially combined
with three levels of dietary protein: 5%, 15%, or 25%.
At 48 days of age subsamples from each group size X
protein combination were assayed for indices of growth
rates and behavioral differences. Indices of neurotransmitter activity and nucleic acid concentrations
were not differentially affected. Animals housed in
the largest group size and maintained on a protein-
augmented diet (25%) were most responsive to their environment as measured by exploratory measures and open-
field tests of emotionality. Observing animals housed
in the smallest group size, body weight, brain weight,
adrenal weight, and pituitary weight varied directly
with protein level in the diet. As group size increased
from groups of 2 to groups of 30, the magnitude of the
relationship between protein level and the above-
specified dependent variables decreased. For the largest
housing groups, there was little relationship between
protein level and any of the morphological and/or
neurochemical indices. The outcomes suggest that increasing social contact attenuates the effects of
protein deficient diets during the early postweaning
development.

Protein Deficiency, Population Density,
and Early Experience

Although characteristically studied independently,
early dietary deficiency and high population density are
often correlated in their natural occurrence. Since
there is some evidence that they affect, in part, the
same physiological processes, it seems fruitful to
investigate their possible interactive effects.

METHODS

Subjects

One hundred and seventy-four male Wistar rats, 21
days of age at the beginning of the experiment, were
assigned randomly to one of nine treatment combinations,
consisting of three group sizes (2, 16, or 30) factorially
combined with three levels of protein-sufficient diet
(5%, 15%, or 25%). The three protein levels constitute
a deprived-, adequate-, and augmented-protein diet, respectively.

Apparatus

Experimental housing consisted of plywood cages
with a mesh floor and top. Cage size was varied pro-
portionally to the group size, with 20 square inches
allocated per animal.

Open-field testing for emotionality utilized a
20 x 20 inch field painted black, with white lines
dividing the floor into 4-inch squares. A 150-watt
bulb was centered 18 inches over the field.

Exploratory behavior and escape-avoidance conditioning utilized a one-way shuttle box with a grid floor.
The start compartment (9 x 12 x 12 inches high) was
separated from the goalbox (15 x 12 x 12 inches high)
by a guillotine door. A 20-watt bulb, mounted on the
rear wall of the start box was the CS. A 110-volt
scrambled shock to the grid floor was the UCS. CS-UCS
and intertrial intervals were controlled by Hunter interval timers. Response latencies were recorded on a
Hunter 0.01-sec timer. Organ weights were measured on
an Ohaus scale calibrated in milligrams.

Procedure

The subjects were housed in the assigned group-diet condition from 21 to 48 days of age. The diet, in the form of mash, was available ad lib for 45 min daily, with water available ad lib.

At 42 days of age, six subjects per group were selected randomly for behavioral testing in the open-field and shuttle-box tasks. One 2-min trial in the open field was conducted on the first and sixth day of testing. On the second day of testing each subject was placed in the shuttle box, with the guillotine door separating the two compartments opened, and permitted to explore the apparatus. The number of midline crossings was tabulated as an index of exploratory behavior. Following the free-exploration session and on the third through fifth day of testing, each animal received 20 trials of escape-avoidance conditioning, using a CS-UCS interval of 5 sec and an intertrial interval ranging from 30 to 60 sec. Throughout this testing period all subjects continued to live under the experimental conditions.

At 48 days of age, six additional subjects were selected randomly for physiological assay. They were weighed and sacrificed, and brains, adrenals, and pituitaries were removed, weighed, and frozen for subsequent analysis. DNA, RNA, and brain protein determinations were performed on brain halves by differential extraction procedures (Wannemacher, Banks, and Wummer, 1965). Norepinehprine and epinephrine concentrations were determined by a trihydroxyindol procedure, modified by microanalyses (Mead and Finger, 1961). AChE activity was estimated by a colorimetric method (Ellman et al., 1961).

Each of the dependent variables was analyzed as a 3 x 3 factorial analysis of variance.

RESULTS

Morphology

Significant (p = 0.01) effects of diet were obtained for all morphological indices of growth. Table I summarizes these effects (summing across all levels of living-group size). It is apparent that a reduced level

TABLE I. Mean Organ Weights as a Function of Dietary Protein

	Protein level		
	5%	15%	25%
Body weight (g)	163.83(48)*	316.22	309.39(2)
Brain weight (g)	1.62(9)	1.78	1.80(1)
Pituitary weight (mg)	5.26(25)	7.01	8.12(14)
Left adrenal weight (mg)	10.01(41)	16.89	17.22(2)

*Denotes percentage difference from mean organ weight under 15% protein diet.

of protein intake (5% vs. 15%) results in reduced body, brain, and adrenal weight; but that a protein-augmented diet (25% vs. 15%) has no impact upon these organ weights. Pituitary weight was reduced for those animals reared on protein-deficient diets and, unlike the other morphological indices, was increased for those animals reared on a protein-augmented diet.

The effects of differential living-group size did not yield significant main effects upon organ weights, but did have a significant (p = 0.01) interactive effect with different combinations of diet. The largest differences in organ weight between the three dietary levels were obtained with those animals housed in groups of 2. Somewhat smaller differences due to dietary differences were obtained with those animals housed in groups of 16. Negligible (not statistically significant) differences in organ weights between the various dietary-protein levels were obtained for those animals housed in groups of 30. The interactive pattern of results suggests that housing animals in near-isolation (2 per cage) enhanced the **differential** consequences of diet, while housing animals in very large groups (30 per cage) minimized the differential consequences of diet.

Neurochemistry

The only significant (p = 0.01) chemical effect of diet was upon concentrations of brain protein, which varied directly with dietary protein levels. Brain protein was not affected by group size. Concentrations of DNA, RNA, epinephrine, and norepinephrine were not differentially affected by any of the experimental conditions, nor was AChE activity.

Behavior

No differences between experimental groups were obtained on the initial open-field trial, either in terms of activity or number of boluses defecated. Significant (p = 0.01) interactive effects were evident on the second trial, following 4 days of escape-avoidance conditioning. Higher levels of dietary protein were associated with greater activity and reduced defecation (low emotional responsiveness). Being housed in larger groups was similarly associated with greater activity and reduced defecation. The two variables combined in a linear fashion, so that the least activity coupled with greatness defecation (high emotionality) was displayed by the animals reared in groups of 2 with a 5% protein diet, and the highest activity level coupled with the least defecation (low emotionality) was displayed by the animals reared in groups of 30 with a 25% protein diet.

Exploratory behavior, as measured by number of midline crossings in the 20-min trial in the shuttle box, followed a pattern similar to that obtained in the open-field test. No differences in escape-avoidance conditioning, either in terms of response latencies or in terms of the number of successful shock-avoidance responses, were obtained between any of the experimental groups.

Discussion

The general morphological effects of a protein-deficient diet upon young animals appears to be highly replicable. The weight differences between the protein-deprived and the normal-protein animals (as expressed in percentages) corresponds fairly closely to those reported previously (Lowry et al., 1962; Howard and Granoff, 1968).

The rank order of impact upon organs—body, adrenals, pituitary, brain—is almost certainly related to the age span during which the animals' diets were manipulated. Dobbing and Widdowen (1965) have suggested that dietary insufficiency has its greatest impact upon those bodily structures which are simultaneously in their period of maximum growth rate.

The interesting outcome of the present experiment is the interactive consequences of different levels of dietary protein with animals housed in different group sizes. Despite Calhoun's (1962) reports of the dire consequences of housing animals under conditions of high population density (which actually appear to be peculiar to his floor-space arrangement), the results of the present experiment suggest that increased living-group size ameliorates, in large part, the consequences of a protein-deficient diet. As has been hypothesized else-where in this conference, it is possible that increased forced social interaction provides a more stimulating environment and that the well-documented effects of protein deficiency are mediated, in part, via reduced organism-environment interaction rather than as a direct dietary consequence.

REFERENCES

Calhoun, J. B., 1962, "Population density in social pathology," Sci. Am. 106:139-150.

Dobbing, J., and Widdowen, E. M., 1965, "The effect of undernutrition and subsequent rehabilitation on myelination of the rat brain as measured by its com-position," Brain 88:357-366.

Ellman, G. L., Courtney, K. D., Andres, V., Jr., and Featherstone, R. M., 1961, "A new and rapid colori-metric determination of acetylcholinesterase activity," Biochem. Pharmacol. 7:88-95.

Howard, E., and Granoff, D. M., 1965, "Effect of neonatal food restriction in mice on brain growth, DNA and cholesterol, and on adult delayed response learning," J. Nutr. 95:111-121.

Lowry, R. S., Pond, W. G., Barnes, R. H., Krook, L., and Loosli, J. K., "Influence of caloric level and protein quality on the manifestations of protein de-ficiency in the young pig," J. Nutr. 78:245-249.

Mead, J. A. R., and Finger, K. F., 1961, "A single
  extraction method for the determination of both
  norepinephrine and seretonin in the brain," Biochem.
  Pharmacol. 6:52-53.
Wannemacher, R. W., Jr., Banks, W. L., Jr., and Wummer,
  W. H., 1965, "Use of a single tissue extract to
  determine cellular protein and nucleic acid concentration and rate of amine acid incorporation," Anal.
  Biochem. 11:320-326.

PROTEIN MALNUTRITION AND COMPLEX LEARNING IN THE CHICKEN

George Collier,* Robert L. Squibb,+ and Paul Hamlin*

*Department of Psychology
+Laboratories of Disease and Environmental Stress
Rutgers University
New Brunswick, New Jersey

Protein malnutrition during periods of rapid growth has long been hypothesized to have deleterious effects on mental capacity (cf. Birch and Gussow, 1970; Scrimshaw and Gordon, 1968). Such a hypothesis is difficult to evaluate since performance is the product of many factors other than intellectual capacity, such as motivation, individual experiential history, vigor, etc. In an attempt to develop an animal model of protein malnutrition that controlled for these various extraneous variables the authors conducted a long series of experiments with chickens and rats, the results of which were negative. That is, it proved impossible under strictly controlled conditions to demonstrate any effect of protein malnutrition which could be attributed to a deficit in capacity. Negative results are **usually not** very interesting. However, these results are presented for their possible heuristic value to future investigators in this area.

The chicken, a precocial bird, was chosen, perhaps unwisely, for the model, since (1) its dietary requirements were well known, (2) it presented no problems of maternal or sibling interaction, (3) it was easy to obtain a genetically homogeneous population, and (4) preliminary experimentation showed that it could learn difficult visual discriminations with relative ease and that there were large individual differences in this capacity.

Dietary conditioning was done by placing the test group on a (utilizable) protein-free diet (ground corn and 5% corn oil) for the two weeks immediately following hatch. This diet produced approximately 30% mortality. The birds were then rehabilitated on the control diet and tested several weeks later. The deficient birds never recovered the control weight. Several variations of this procedure were tried to heighten the effects of malnutrition.

The test problem chosen was designed to separate motivational from intellectual factors. It consisted of teaching the bird to discriminate between two visual stimuli (horizontal and vertical stripes in most cases). In addition to the two visual stimuli a third key was used. The bird was required to "set up" the problem by making a series of responses (usually 15) on this center key. Completion of this ratio produced the problem. A correct choice was followed by 15 sec access to food. An incorrect response was followed by an 8 sec blackout. Following either of these cases the center key was again available for setting up the next trial. After the bird had reached a criterion of 95% correct choices, the problem was reversed; that is, correct and incorrect stimuli were interchanged. Each time the bird reached criterion the stimuli were again reversed. This stimulus reversal problem controlled for any possible sensory deficits resulting from malnutrition. Two measures were obtained: (1) the rate of problem presentation and (2) the percentage of correct choices over successive reversals.

Looking at the mean number of errors to criterion over successive reversals, it was clear that\there were no differences between groups. Since the malnourished group had a somewhat slower rate of problem presentation, the birds were sorted into fast and slow groups and Figure 1 presents the results of this segregation. Again, there were no differences. Thus, the rate of problem presentation, a measure of motivation, was not correlated with ability to learn the discrimination. The results of a different version of this experiment are presented in Figure 2. Three groups, normal diet, rehabilitated low-protein diet, and a concurrent low-protein diet were used. These results show that concurrent malnourishment also did not effect reversal learning performance.

As previously reported, normal birds responded at higher rates on FR schedules. Since malnourished birds may have a lower response-rate ceiling than normals,

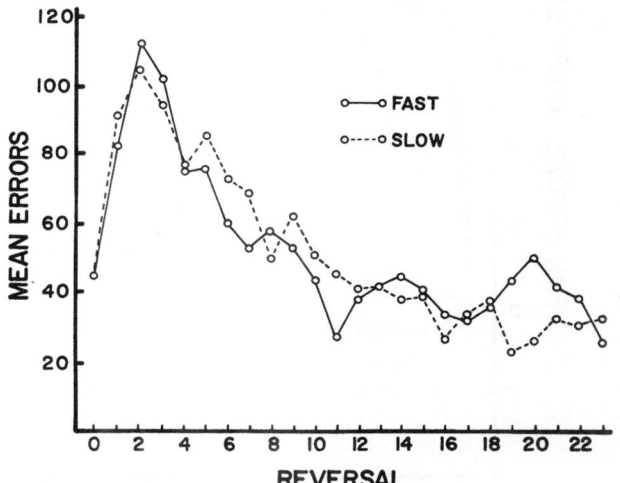

FIGURE 1. Mean errors to criterion as a function
of reversal for fast and slow responding
birds.

G. COLLIER, R. L. SQUIBB, AND P. HAMLIN

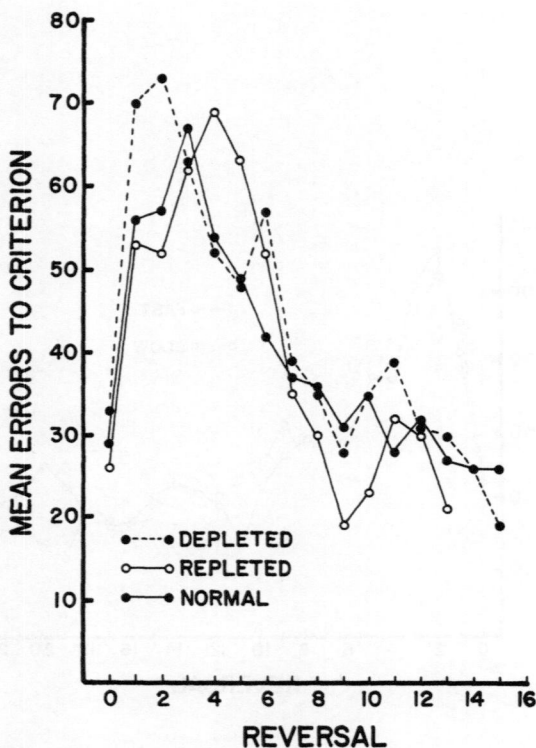

FIGURE 2. Mean errors to criterion as a function of
          reversals in normal, repleted, and protein-
          depleted groups. The depleted group was
          maintained on a low-protein diet from birth.
          The repleted group was rehabilitated after
          being maintained on a low-protein diet the
          first three weeks of life. The normal con-
          trol group was fed a standard diet.

three groups of birds were tested in variable interval
schedules which produced lower levels of responding.
Again, the same results were obtained (Figure 3).
Normal birds responded at higher rates. Thus, it
appears that there was a difference in vigor or motivation between the malnourished and normal birds but
no differences in ability to learn complex visual discrimination.

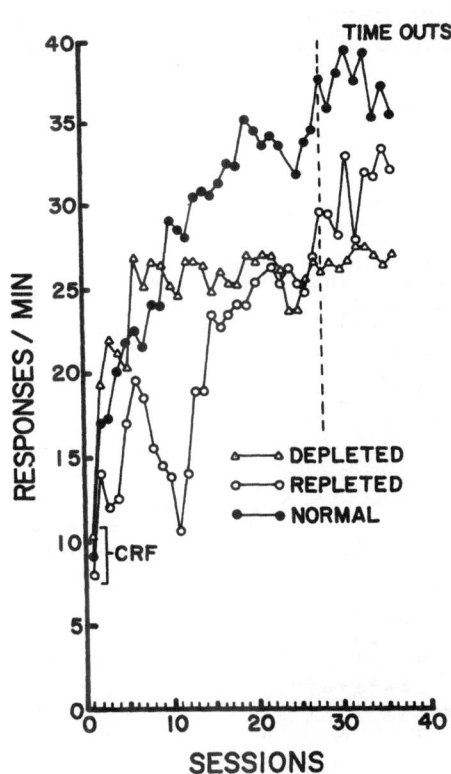

FIGURE 3. Mean response rates for normal, repleted, and
          protein-depleted on a VI 1 minute schedule.
          To the right of the dashed line, four-second
          time-out periods were superimposed on the
          variable interval interval 1 minute schedule.

As a final sample of our attempts to measure the effects of malnutrition on mental capacity, we tested the hypothesis that malnourished birds' capacity to inhibit responding might be impaired. Two experiments will be briefly reported. The first used a multiple schedule, VI 1 minute-extinction. Thus, a comparison between groups responding during extinction was possible. Various levels of deprivation were used. The results shown in Figures 4 and 5 show that there were rate differences in the malnourished birds but no differences in number of extraneous responses during the extinction component of the schedule, and thus no evidence for differential ability to inhibit. Finally, malnourished and control birds were tested on DRL (differential reinforcement of low rates). Here again, it was impossible to show any differences as a function of dietary history.

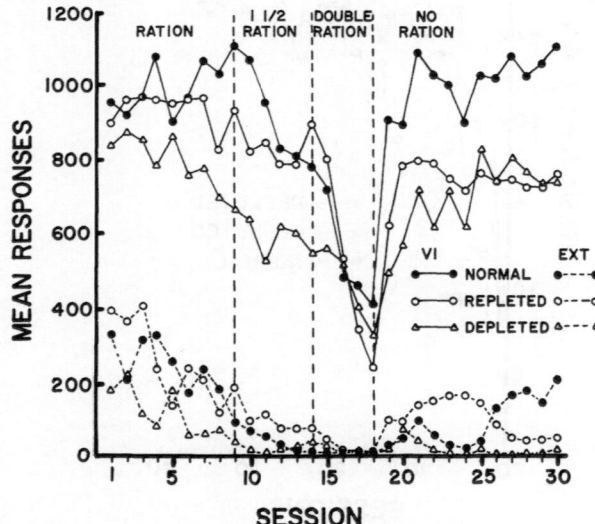

FIGURE 4. Mean absolute number of responses as a
          function of the sessions for variable
          interval 1 minute (VI) and extinction (EXT)
          components of the multiple schedule for
          normal, repleted, and protein-depleted groups
          of birds in Multi VI 1 minute extinction.

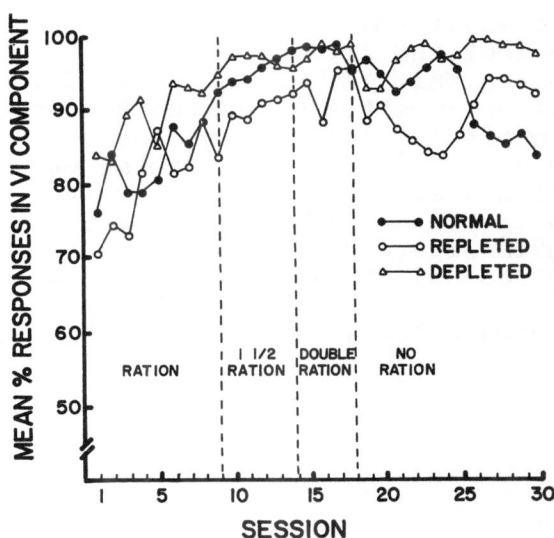

FIGURE 5. Mean percent total responses during the variable interval 1 minute component of the
multiple schedule for the three groups of
chickens in Multi VI 1 minute extinction.

It is very difficult to draw conclusions from
negative results, since there are any number of possible
reasons why the results were obtained, but it seems
likely from the data presented above that it is difficult
to produce deficits in ability to perform complex tasks
in chickens by means of protein malnourishment, a conclusion that seems correct for a widening number of
species.

There is a second effect of concurrent dietary
protein levels which may account for some of the performance differences noted in malnourished populations.
The level of spontaneous activity (observed in running
wheels) varies with the ratios of protein, fat, and
carbohydrate in the diet (Collier and Squibb, 1967).
The levels of running as a function of three levels of
protein, L (5.6%), N (20.0%), and H (59.6%) are shown

in Figure 6. Two environments were used, one in which
the animals were isolated from laboratory stimulation
and one in which the animals were maintained in the
colony. It is clear from **these results that rats maintained on low-protein** diets show high levels of spontaneous activity while **high-protein diets, under some cir-**
cumstances, depressed activity. Growth curves for these
animals compared with animals without access to running
wheels are shown in Figure 7. Activity depressed growth
rate of normally fed animals (see also Collier, 1970),
increased growth rate of animals fed high protein, and
did not affect animals fed low protein. The effect of

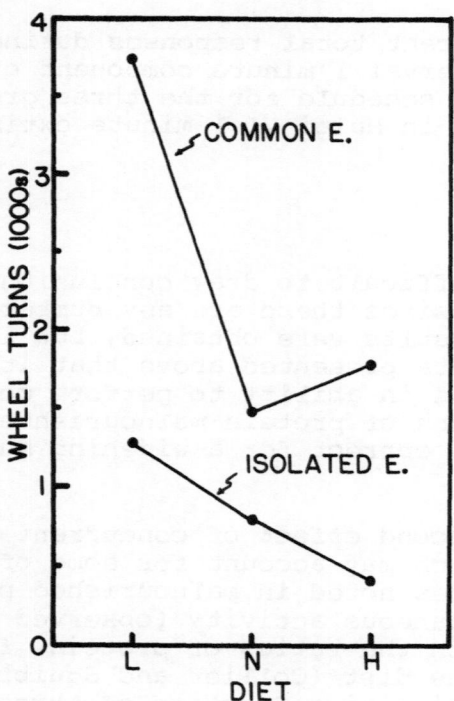

FIGURE 6. Wheel turns per day as a function of dietary
           levels of protein and environment.

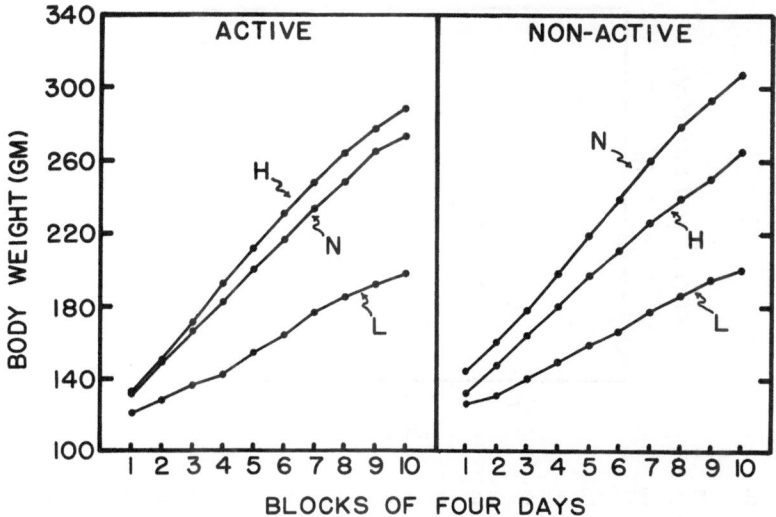

FIGURE 7. Growth rate as a function of dietary levels
         of protein and activity.

activity on animals eating high-protein diets, an
effect we have often observed, is interesting from the
point of view of how an adequate diet is defined. If,
as often is the case, growth rate is used to determine
"optimum" diets, it suggests that the caged-sedentary
rat is a poor model for dietary studies. Some of these
differences in growth rate can be accounted for in
terms of food intake, shown in Figure 8. Imbalanced
diets reduced food intake. Activity depressed food
intake of diets containing low or normal amounts of
protein (see Collier, 1970) and stimulated intake of
diets containing high levels of protein. Finally, for
these data, the effect on body temperatures of these
diets should be noted (Figure 9). Body temperature
proved to be an inverse function of level of protein.
This effect was independent of activity, since it
occurred in both the active and inactive animals.

     In an attempt to assess which component, protein,
carbohydrate, or fat, was responsible for the changes
in level of activity, an experiment similar to the
preceding was performed in which all three components

G. COLLIER, R. L. SQUIBB, AND P. HAMLIN

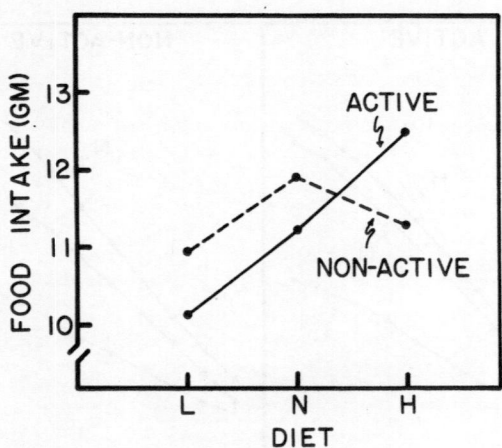

FIGURE 8. Food intake as a function of dietary levels
of protein and activity.

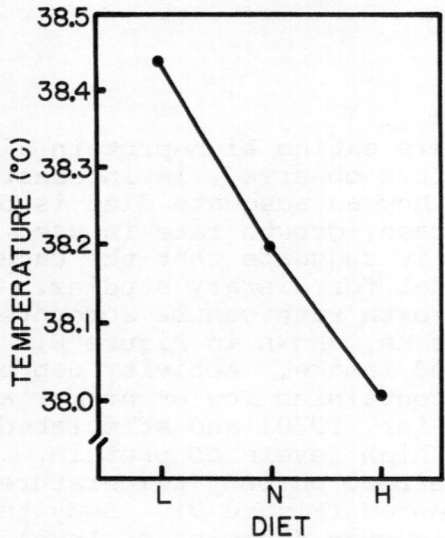

FIGURE 9. Body temperature as a function of dietary
levels of protein.

of the diet were varied. The main results are presented
in Figure 10. These correlational results suggest that
it is the ratio of percentage of protein to energy in
the diet which is associated with different levels of
activity. Following this lead a further experiment was
done in which fat, carbohydrate, and protein were held
constant, but in which a single amino acid, lysine, was
present in deficient quantities in the otherwise adequate
test diet. The level of lysine was used as a limiting
factor for protein synthesis. The growth curves for the
test diet, a **pair-fed control group, and the ad lib-fed**
control group are shown in Figure 11. The low-lysine
diet (sesame oil meal) resulted in a lower growth rate.
Figure 12, on the other hand, shows that there was a
fourfold increase in activity over the period of increasing deficiency. A **pair-fed group run at a later**
date showed that this increase in activity was not solely
the result of weight loss, but mainly due to the deficiency.

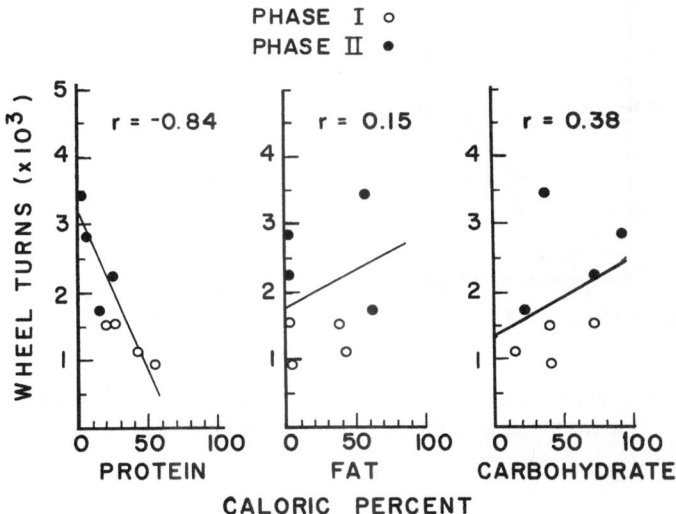

FIGURE 10. Wheel turns as a function the caloric percent
of protein, fat, or carbohydrate in the diet.

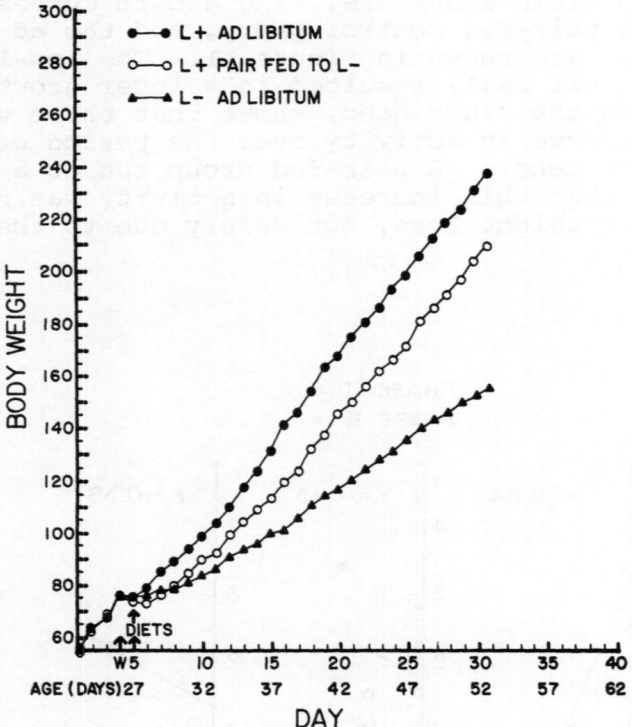

FIGURE 11. Growth rate as a function of adequate and
          inadequate levels of lysine in the diet.

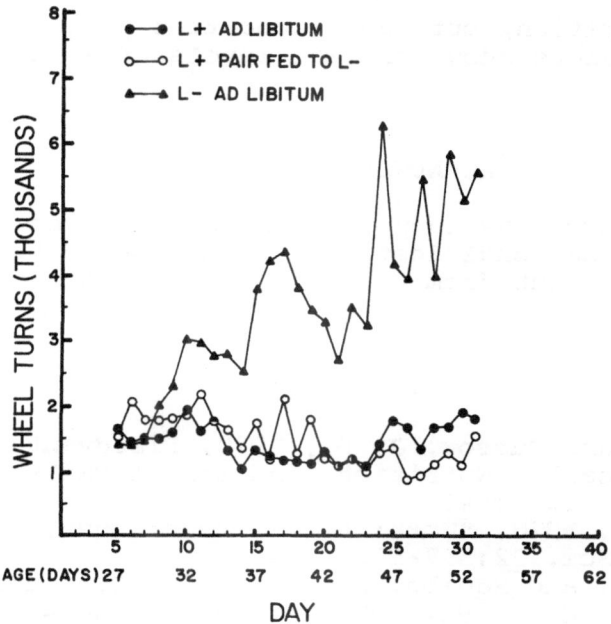

FIGURE 12. Wheel turns as a function of adequate and
          inadequate levels of lysine in the diet.

The results of these experiments show that the level
of protein in the diet of a growing animal has a large
effect on his level of spontaneous activity. Animals
fed low-protein diets show large increases in activity.
It is tempting to conjecture that some of the performance
deficits reported for protein-malnourished populations may
arise from hyperactivity induced by their poor diet. If
the data from the concurrently malnourished chickens in
the learning of a complex discrimination can be extrapo-
lated, showing no discrimination performance deficit as a
result of a low-protein diet, performance deficits would
have to result from an interaction of the hyperactivity
with the task rather than from a deficit in capacity. For
example, hyperactive children are notorious problems in the
school situation. Such interactions remain to be explored.

In summary, we have been unable to show deficits in
intellectual capacity resulting from prior or concurrent

protein malnutrition, but have found that growing animals fed such diets show abnormal levels of spontaneous
activity.

ACKNOWLEDGMENT

    This research was supported in part by grant HD-
03279 from the National Institute of Health, Bethesda,
Maryland and a grant from the Nutrition Foundation,
New York, N. Y.

REFERENCES

Birch, H. G., and Gussow, J. D., 1970, Disadvantaged
    Children. Health, Nutrition, and School Failure. Har-
    court Brace, New York.
Collier, G. H., 1970, "Work: A weak reinforcer," Trans.
    N. Y. Acad. Sci. 32:557-576.
Collier, G. H., and Squibb, R. L., 1967, "Diet and
    activity," J. Comp. Physiol. Psychol. 64:409-413.
Scrimshaw, N. S., and Gordon, J. E., 1968, Malnutrition,
    Learning, and Behavior, M. I. T. Press, Cambridge,
    Mass.

LEARNING IN CHRONICALLY PROTEIN-DEPRIVED RATS

Gerald Turkewitz

Department of Pediatrics
Albert Einstein College of Medicine
        and
Department of Psychology
Hunter College, New York, N.Y.

I am going to describe findings which are somewhat
at variance with the findings that others have presented.
Cowley and Griesel (1959, 1963) reported differences in
the learning ability of protein-deprived and adequately
nourished rats. In a number of the presentations made
today it has been pointed out that motivational differences, motor differences, and attentional differences
can all affect learning without necessarily reflecting
any differences in learning ability per se. In fact,
it was rather elegantly demonstrated that when proper
attention is paid to such factors, it is extremely
difficult to find differences in learning ability between well nourished and poorly nourished animals. However, it should be noted that Cowley and Griesel's studies differed from those reported today not just with
respect to the nature of the findings but with regard to
the nature of the animals studied as well. That is, the
animals which Cowley and Griesel found to be most deficient in learning were protein-deprived animals born to
and reared by animals which had themselves been protein-
deprived. It is therefore possible that the differences
in results obtained by Cowley and Griesel and by the
participants in this conference do not represent differences in the niceties of controlling factors other than
learning but rather represent differences in the consequences of acute episodes of malnutrition as opposed to
chronic intergenerational protein deficiencies. With

this possibility in mind I would like to discuss the
learning of a group of rats which had been chronically
protein-deprived for from 6 to 8 generations. The research that I am going to discuss was carried out in
collaboration with Drs. R. J. C. Stewart and the late
Herbert G. Birch. The animals we studied are those
which Dr. Stewart described in detail earlier.

As was pointed out earlier, one of the problems
with which one is confronted in attempting to assess
the effects of protein deficiencies upon intellectual
functioning is the problem of insuring that differences
between well and poorly nourished animals are not a
function of differences in either motor ability or motivation. For example, it is clear that time measures
might not be very useful if malnutrition affected vigor
of response; similarly it is obvious that the same food
reward might have different incentive value for well
nourished animals and animals who are either currently
malnourished or who had a history of malnutrition. Less
obvious, but equally important, even treatments not
directly related to the animal's nutritional history can
have important consequences for the animal's behavior in
a learning situation. It has, for example, been pointed
out today that well and poorly nourished animals do not
respond to electric shock in the same manner. We believe
that we have developed a technique for testing the effects
of protein deficiency on certain aspects of learning
ability which avoids some of the difficulties associated
with studying this problem. Our technique involves a
modification of the jumping-stand technique.

Many years ago, Karl Lashley (1930) developed a
technique for testing discrimination learning in rats.
The technique involved having rats jump from an elevated
stand through one of two doors on which were displayed
various patterns. One of the patterns was "correct" and
one "incorrect." The door on which the "incorrect" figure was mounted was latched so that if the animals jumped
at the incorrect pattern he would bump his nose and fall
into a net mounted below the doors. If he jumped at the
correct pattern the door swung open and he landed on a
platform on which was placed a small food reward. We
thought that the food reward might not be essential to
training the animals. Therefore, to avoid the problem
of differential incentive effects of food on the two
types of rats, we simply omitted the use of food as an
incentive from the procedure.

The procedure which we utilized consisted of pushing the animals off the platform if they did not jump spontaneously. If they jumped to the wrong door they would bump their noses and fall. If they jumped to the correct door, the door would swing open and they would be "home safe." Under these circumstances the rats readily learned to jump from the elevated stand through one of the two unlatched doors. Having determined that the jumping-stand technique could be utilized even without the typical deprivation and food reward procedure, we set about devising a battery of visual discrimination tasks of graded difficulty for the rat. Previous investigations (Lashley, 1930) have indicated that a black-white discrimination is quite easy for the rat. Horizontal-vertical stripe discrimination is relatively more difficult and still more difficult is circle-triangle discrimination. We thought that by using a graded battery consisting of these three discrimination tasks, it would be possible to do several things. First, we would be able to determine whether or not we had, in fact, devised a procedure which reduced or eliminated any differences in learning attributable to motivational differences. We were hoping that the well nourished and the poorly nourished animals would respond similarly on the simplest discrimination, the black-white discrimination. If they were to do that it would be possible to argue that since the incentive does not change from discrimination to discrimination, any differences found between the groups on subsequent discrimination training could not be due to a motivational difference. Similarly, since the motor behavior involved in all three discriminations is identical, any differences between groups could not be readily attributable to differences in motor ability.

When we examine the data for learning the black-white discrimination, we see that the well nourished (B diet) and the poorly nourished (A diet) animals do not differ with regard to either the percentage of animals reaching the criteria for learning (eight correct responses in a row) or the number of trials required to reach criterion. As can be seen in the first figure, 100% of the well nourished and almost 95% of the poorly nourished animals reached the criterion. Furthermore, the rate of learning in the two groups was quite similar, with all of the animals who learned the discrimination doing so within 50 trials. Neither the differences between the percentage of animals in the two groups achieving criterion nor that in rate of learning was significant.

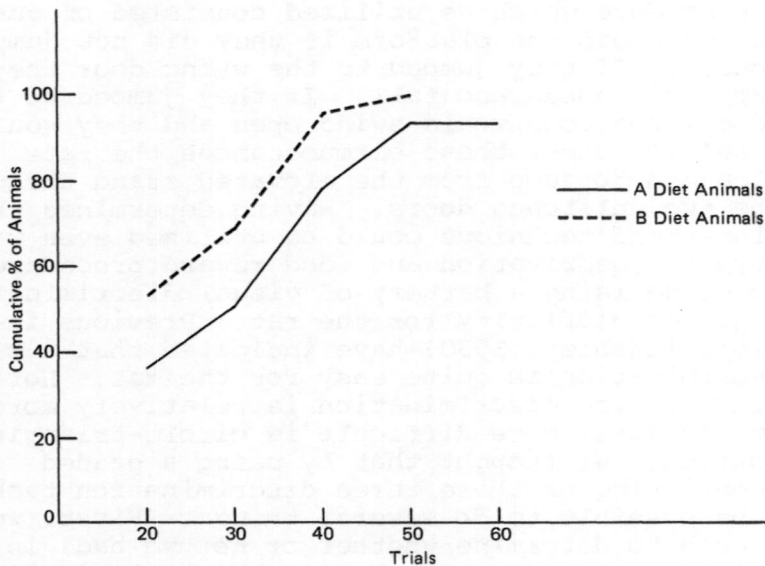

FIGURE 1. Number of trials to reach criterion for
solution of black-white discrimination.

Before discussing the results of the next two
discriminations I would like to point out that because
the three discriminations chosen for study form a series
of graded difficulty, the procedure which we utilized
involved eliminating an animal from further study if it
failed (within 110 trials) to reach the criterion for
learning on an earlier problem. That is, the animal who
failed on the black-white discrimination did not move on
to the next discrimination, but was eliminated from
further testing. Similarly, animals who failed to learn
the horizontal-vertical discrimination did not move on
to the circle-triangle task. In this way we were always
dealing with animals with equal histories of success at
the start at each discrimination. It should be noted
that the percentage of animals achieving criterion represents the percentage of animals starting a given
problem who solved that problem.

If we look at Figure 2, we see that the well
nourished animals continue to do quite well on the
horizontal-vertical discrimination with 95% of the

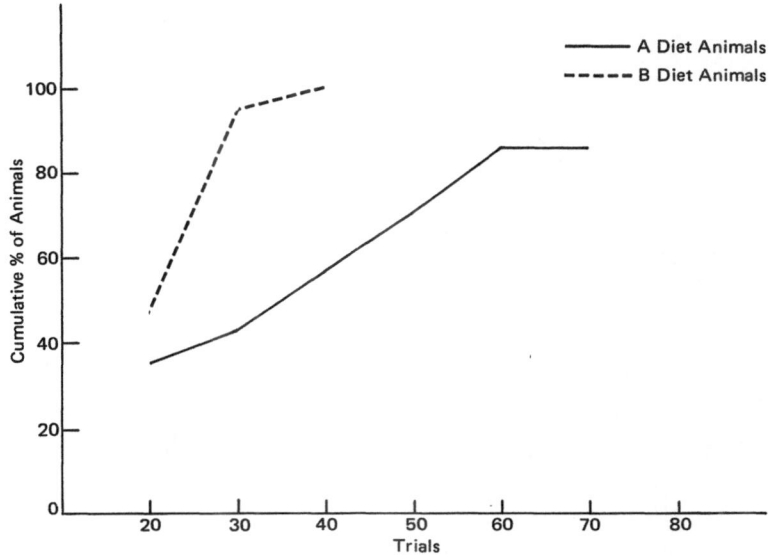

FIGURE 2. Number of trials to reach criterion for
          solution of horizontal-vertical discrimination.

animals learning the discrimination within 30 trials and
100% reaching criterion within 40 trials. In marked
contrast to this is the performance of the poorly
nourished animals. Inspection of the figure reveals
that by 40 trials (the point at which all of the well
nourished animals had mastered the problem) only a
little over half of the A diet animals had reached
criterion. Furthermore only 86% of animals in this
group ever reach criterion.

    Examination of Figure 3 indicates that the circle-
triangle discrimination was indeed the most difficult
discrimination for the rats; only 84% of the well
nourished and 50% of the previously successful poorly
nourished animals mastered the discrimination. As was
the case for the horizontal-vertical discrimination,
differences between the groups with regard to both
percentage of animals solving the discrimination and
rate of solution are readily apparent. Analysis of the

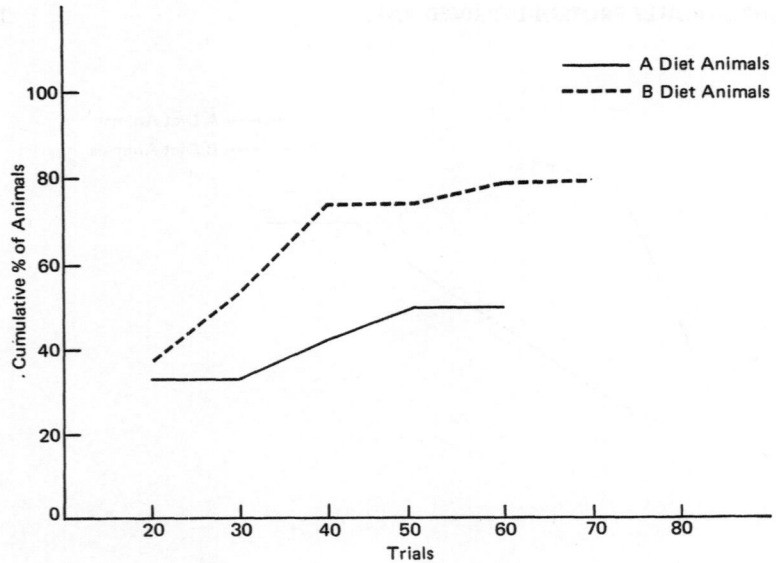

FIGURE 3. Number of trials to reach criterion for
         solution of circle-triangle discrimination.

data reveals significant differences between the groups
both with regard to the proportion of animals learning
the discrimination and the time taken by those who did
learn to reach criterion.

    If we examine the performance of the two types of
animals on the entire battery of discriminations,
differences between the groups are even more marked
than when we look at the results of individual discriminations. As may be seen in Figure 4, while only
40% of the malnourished animals solve all three problems,
84% of the well nourished animals do so. Furthermore
while over 60% of the well nourished rats solve all
three problems within 40 trials, only slightly more than
7% of the poorly nourished animals do so.

    We believe that the differences in the performances
of the well and poorly nourished animals represent clear
and dramatic evidence of differences in learning ability

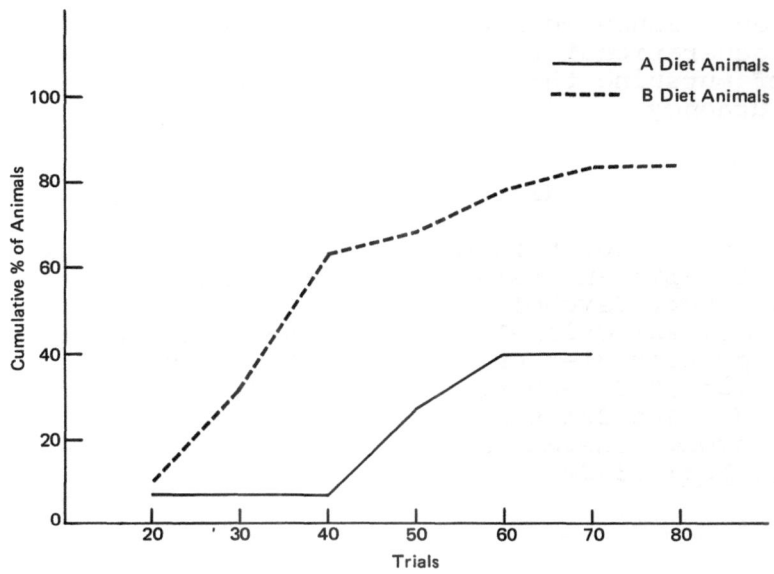

FIGURE 4. Number of trials to reach criterion for
          solution of black-white horizontal-vertical
          and circle-triangle discrimination.

and in speed of learning. We further believe that these
differences cannot be ascribed to motivational differences or to differences in motor ability. Since
there was no difference between groups on the easiest
discrimination, and since the easiest discrimination
and the more difficult discriminations all require
identical motor performances while utilizing identical
incentives, it is difficult to see how group differences
can be the result of either of these factors.

      We therefore believe that the discrepancy in re-
sults between the clearcut difference which we have
found as contrasted with the failure by others to find
differences in the learning of well and poorly nourished
animals may well be a function of differences between
animals with an intergenerational history of poor nutrition and those suffering a more acute single-generation

malnutrition. Since much of human malnutrition is of
this intergenerational type we believe that the importance of pursuing this type of model therefore assumes
increased urgency.

REFERENCES

Lashley, K. S., 1930, "The mechanism of vision. 1. A
  method for rapid analysis of pattern-vision in the
  rat," J. Genet. Psychol. 37:353-460.
Cowley, J. J., and Griesel, R. D., 1959, "Some effects
  of a low protein diet on a first filial generation
  of white rats," J. Genet. Psychol., 95:187-201.
Cowley, J. J., and Griesel, R. D., 1963, "The development of second-generation low-protein rats," J. Genet.
  Psychol., 103:233-242.

CONCLUDING REMARKS

Myron Winick

Director, Institute of Human Nutrition

Columbia University College of Physicians
and Surgeons

New York, N.Y.

Unfortunately, one scientist who participated in
the organization of this symposium is no longer with us,
Dr. Herbert Birch. Dr. Birch was a pioneer in this field.
Most of us were privileged to have known him for a long
time, and we are all saddened by his passing.

What I thought I would do is attempt to synthesize
some of the complex data which we discussed today, and
to indicate directions in which these data might move us
tomorrow. Three or four years ago, I attended a series
of conferences sponsored by the National Institutes of
Health on nutrition and its relation to mental development
and brain growth. It is interesting to see the kinds of
concerns that we have now and to compare them with the
kinds of concerns we had then.

At that time much emphasis was placed on descriptive
efforts. We were attempting to describe either at the
biochemical level or at the functional level what happens
during malnutrition in the early period of life, and
whether or not the effects of malnutrition are reversible.
A host of effects has been described: you have heard about
them today. In the animal model the concern was both the
isolation of malnutrition and the kinds of measurements
we were making, be they biological or psychological. I

think it is fair to say that at that time in animal
experiments, the concern was much more: what do these
measurements mean? It was assumed that we could
isolate malnutrition in the animal; that was the reason
for using an animal model, since it was so difficult to
isolate in the human.

It is interesting for me to see the concern shift
and evolve to question: can we really isolate malnutrition from the rest of the environment of the animal
using the kinds of techniques that we have been using?
We saw today that all kinds of changes occur when one
attempts to isolate an animal. The interplay between
the mother and the infant pup changes, or the relationship of the pups to each other may change; and so we
are not now as complacent in our isolation of the
nutritional variable.

On the other hand, it would seem to me, as an
outsider looking in, that the psychological group is
now using techniques and methods which appear to be
more objective measures than those used before. So
there has been, in my judgment, a sort of reversal in
terms of asking the kinds of questions that one can ask
using functional parameters. One would hope that the
group studying function will be as successful in dis-
secting out these other variables and trying to isolate
the nutritional components as they have been in identifying the kinds of functional parameters to study.

From the biochemical standpoint, we have followed
the psychological group by shifting directions, but
nowhere near as fast, so that we also assumed that what
we were producing was malnutrition, pure malnutrition,
and that we did not have to worry about variables in
animals. And it is also becoming obvious to us that we
may not be studying malnutrition alone. So work has
begun on examining the biochemical changes which are
induced by the kinds of interactive situations described.

Many of the people interested in malnutrition at
the biochemical level have switched gears for what I
consider a fascinating reason; that is, that malnutrition has provided a model by which one is able to
study certain basic biochemical phenomena involved in
growth of organs and the central nervous system. Therefore what has happened is that concern for the purity of
the stimulus has decreased, because what one really

wanted is growth retardation, which could be reversed
by refeeding; therefore one was not terribly worried about
whether this growth retardation was due to malnutrition
interacting with the environment.

The question in fact that concerns the people
interested in the biochemistry of the central
nervous system has shifted a bit, and I would hope that
a foundation such as this could help develop an interaction between the people who want to study the purity
of the stimulus at the biochemical level and those who
want to study it at the psychological level. One would
like to see these kinds of work going on in parallel.
I do not think there is a great deal of it at present.
There are a few laboratories, but we certainly need more
of this kind of work.

From today's presentations, it would appear that
the descriptive data are continuing to be gathered.
But regarding parameters, I think the exciting prospect
on the horizon is developing methods of biochemically
diagnosing and following the course of malnutrition,
specifically with reference to fetal malnutrition.
There are now a number of biochemical tests which are
beginning to be developed using maternal white cells,
maternal serum, amniotic fluid, and maternal urine,
which are beginning to tell us how the fetus is growing.
These tests seem to change during altered nutritional
states. And interestingly enough, this investigation
has been encouraged by the changes that were found in
the tissues of malnourished animals.

For example, Dr. Sigulem in Brazil has reported that
the activity of alkaline RNase, the enzyme I showed you
that goes up in the brain of malnourished animals, is
markedly elevated in the serum of malnourished children,
and that after two weeks of intensive therapy this drops
back to normal levels. In further studies that Dr. Sigulem
has done it would appear that this is a very sensitive
indicator of nutritional status, probably not specific,
but sensitive, at least as far as we can tell. Dr.
Metcalfe, working in Mexico and in Oklahoma, has shown
that the activities of certain enzymes in the white
cells of malnourished women are different and that these
activities correlate with the growth rate and the ultimate size of the infant.

So we are expanding our body of knowledge in regard
to pregnancy by using some of the biochemical parameters

which we have learned from the changes that occur in
animal tissues. This has application to the pregnant
population in a clinically helpful way by determining
how and when to intervene with whatever types of intervention possible.

I think that there is no question that the use of
the animal model and biochemical, physiological, and
psychological techniques all have added a great deal
to what we know at the present time. There is also no
question that the really important kinds of problems
that all of us are ultimately interested in are problems
that are going to be dealt with tomorrow, in terms of
the specific effects that these variables have on the
functioning of children.

CLINICAL AND FOLLOW-UP STUDIES RELATED TO MENTAL FUNCTIONING OF MALNOURISHED CHILDREN

SOCIAL ANTECEDENTS AND CORRELATES OF PRESCHOOL

MALNUTRITION IN CAMBRIDGE, MASSACHUSETTS

Ernesto Pollitt

Department of Nutrition and Food Sciences
Massachusetts Institute of Technology
Cambridge, Massachusetts
        and
Eleanor Paradise

Department of Psychology
Emmanuel College
Boston, Massachusetts

INTRODUCTION

The purpose of this paper is to present preliminary data on a study conducted in Cambridge, Massachusetts by staff from the Department of Nutrition and Food Science at MIT on the identification of causal determinants of preschool malnutrition among low-income families.

MALNUTRITION IN MASSACHUSETTS

Data from the Massachusetts State Nutrition Survey (1972) showed that the curves for mean weights and heights of children below six years of age fall between the 25th and 50th percentiles of the Boston Growth Standards. Moreover, approximately three times as many children were below the third percentile as would be expected.

A survey we conducted at MIT of 99 Caucasian children attending the Pediatric Out-Patient Clinic at Cambridge Hospital during a 5 week period in 1972 and of the medical records of 145 children followed at one

of the seven Neighborhood Health Centers in Cambridge,
found 60 children under the 10th percentile. This
represents 24% of the 244 cases, 14% above the expected
number. Twenty children, or 13%, from the Health Center
were below the 3rd percentile for both height and weight.
Poor nutrition is agreed as the major cause of retarded
growth and development in infancy and early childhood.
The significance of these data on stunted growth is that
it suggests a prevalence of malnutrition sufficient to
cause considerable concern.

Evidence has been accumulating that more often than
not malnutrition is no simple result of lack of purchasing
power, although it is clear that income is a determinant
of community nutritional status (Stim et al., 1972).
Explanations based on ignorance of food values are like-
wise insufficient. Studies done in developing countries
and some information from nutrition studies done in this
country, including the Ten State Nutrition Survey and
clinical reports of children diagnosed as failure to
thrive, support a multifactorial etiology of malnutrition
(Talbot and Howell, 1971).

The development of effective treatment and preventive
programs of malnutrition will clearly depend on the
availability of evidence on the important determinants of
this condition. At present, information concerning determinants and course of malnutrition in a U.S. urban
industrial community is insufficient. The need for such
information is evident.

PURPOSE

The purpose of the study which we at the Department
of Nutrition and Food Science at MIT have been conducting
is to examine ecologically the complex of causation in
community malnutrition giving primary emphasis to social
and behavioral factors. The study is based on a comparison of families with and without a malnourished preschool child in the city of Cambridge. The data presented
here are from an exploratory study conducted for the
development of methods and the refinement of hypotheses.

VARIABLES

The premise of the ecological approach used is that
the cause and course of malnutrition results from the
interaction of multiple sources within a host and its
environment (Gordon and Pollitt, 1973). Thus the vari-

ables we are investigating are of three kinds: (1) host, (2) environment, and (3) agent.

Host factors are those which increase or decrease vulnerability or susceptibility to malnutrition, modifying the effects of environmental factors. Physical, biological, and social environmental factors are considered by the ecological model. However, in U.S. urban industrial centers where malnutrition is primarily a man-made problem, social factors are the most significant environmental determinant of community malnutrition. Hence, emphasis is being given to social environmental factors. The agent, or the immediate antecedent cause of the disease process, is, in malnutrition, insufficient food, or deficiency in one or more essential nutrients.

The specific variables studied are listed in Table I. The selection of these variables followed an exhaustive review of available literature on social and behavioral factors associated with malnutrition and related public health problems.

METHOD

Population

The sample for the exploratory phase is drawn from children 1 through 4 years of age attending the Outpatient Pediatric Clinic at Cambridge Hospital. Despite methodological disadvantages, this procedure is satisfactory for pilot purposes and it was chosen because of its practicality.

Twelve- to 59-month-old children below the 3rd percentile in both height and weight were chosen as index cases. Selection criteria required that index subjects had normal full-term births, weighed at least 2500 g at birth, and present no evidence of physical disability, severe mental retardation, or brain damage. Further, following an exhaustive physical examination and laboratory tests, all cases presenting signs of underlying disease were excluded. No restrictions on sex or ethnic backgrounds were made.

Control children were matched with index children for age ($\pm$3 months), sex, and color. Selection criteria also required that they have had normal birth and subsequent development, were over the 25th percentile in height and weight and had no sibling with past or present signs of growth retardation.

TABLE I. Environmental, Agent, and Host Variables Selected for Study

Environmental (social)	Agent	Host
1. Family income	1. Family food purchasing practices	1. Age
2. Family size	2. Child's diet	2. Sex
3. Household density	3. Family's meal patterns	3. Medical history
4. Maternal		4. Eating behavior
1.4.1. Age		
1.4.2. Education		
1.4.3. Occupation		
1.4.4. Competence		
5. History of family changes		
1.5.1. Marital		
1.5.2. Mobility		
1.5.3. Household composition		
1.5.4. Health		

Procedure

Collection of social and behavioral data involved a three month series of in-depth, semistructured 2 hr interviews with the caretaker of the child and behavioral observations of the child, siblings, and mother. Interviews and observations regarding each of the variables already presented were conducted in the home by public health nurses with a master's degree in child psychiatric nursing.

This presentation will focus on data concerning maternal age, history of significant family changes and crises, maternal psychiatric history, and child's ordinal position in the 12 index cases whose studies have already been completed. Similarities in the relation among the variables selected in the 12 families suggesting the existance of two different types of family patterns within this group will be discussed. No data on controls will be presented here.

The age range for the group of 12 was from 12 to 51 months with a mean of 33 months; mean height and weight age were 24 to 19 months, respectively. The large time differential between chronological age and height and weight age show the considerable degree of growth retardation among these children.

Ten of the twelve children were white; two were black. The relatively small number of black children matched the proportion of blacks in the Cambridge community. There were eight males and four females; the reason for this sex ratio is not yet clear.

Table II presents the income of 11 families as reported by the mothers interviewed. Data are not available in one case because of the interviewee's reluctance to supply this information. Yearly income was estimated from the family's account of their monthly income which allegedly represented the total sum from all sources. The table also presents the poverty levels, by family size, used by the Social Security Administration for nonfarm families. The column on differences between yearly income and poverty levels shows that among the 11 families for whom quantitative reports are available, 7 had incomes higher than the poverty level. The range in the reported income shows that the differences in the economic status of the high- and low-income families was of considerable magnitude.

TABLE II. Estimated Income of Eleven Index Families

Identification number	Family size	Yearly income	Poverty level[a]	Difference Y.I.-P.L.
01	3	NA	$3450	Estimated above
02	4	$7920	$4200	+ 3720
03	2	$2251	$2725	- 474
04	2	$2592	$2725	- 133
05	7	$5448	$6200	- 752
06	6	$6000	$5550	+ 450
07	4	$7320	$4200	+ 3120
08	4	$2640	$4200	- 1560
09	9	$7824	$7500	+ 324
10	2	$3588[b]	$2725	+ 863
11	3	$5808[c]	$3450	+ 2358
12	6	$8592	$5550	+ 3042

a   January 9, 1973 Social Security Administration estimate for nonfarm families, based on 1970 U.S. Census Data.

b   plus unknown amount from 5 day/week half-time baby sitting.

c   plus unknown amount from common-law husband.

Table III presents data on the child's ordinal position, mother's marital status, age, and education as well as the source of economic subsistence at the time of the child's birth. The data show the following similarities: (1) seven of the children were their mother's only child; (2) four of these mothers were single and five were younger than 21 years of age at the time of the child's birth; (3) the remaining five children were born to women over 21 years of age who were more likely to be married at the child's birth. Three who were late-borns (4th- to 7th-born) had mothers over 30 years of age at the time of the child's birth.

In order to combine these data, maternal age was divided into three ranges: (a) 21 years of age or younger, (b) 22-29, and (c) 30 years old or older. Marital status was categorized as single or married; the two separated and divorced women were included in the category of single

TABLE III. Descriptive Data at Child's Birth: Ordinal Position; Mother's Marital Status, Age, and Education; Economic Source of Subsistence

Identification number	Ordinal position	Mother's marital status	Mother's age	Mother's education	Economic source of subsistence
01	only child	single	19	12th	self-support
02	only child	single	14	7th	welfare
03	only child	single	20	vocational school	welfare
04	only child	married	28	12th	husband's work
05	6th	married	32	11th	welfare
06	4th	married	33	11th	husband's work
07	only child	separated	22	11th	welfare
08	2nd	married	22	12th	welfare
09	7th	married	31	12th	husband's work
10	only child	single	20	12th	welfare
11	only child	divorced	21	12th	welfare
12	3rd	married	23	college	husband's work

because they did not have a marital or common-law relationship at the time the children were born. Ordinal
position was divided into three subgroups: (a) single
child; (b) 2nd- or 3rd-born; (c) 4th- or later-born.
Education of the mother was excluded from any further
calculations because of its small variance and its
apparent random association with the remaining variables.

To determine whether there were underlying patterns
in the data on economic source, maternal age, marital
status, and child's ordinal position, all those cases
with identical values in three of the four variables
listed were identified and grouped together. Table IV
presents in summary form the data for all 12 cases
grouped in this manner. Two patterns are observed.
The first, which includes 50% of the children, is characterized by an only child of a woman who is young (21
years old or younger), single, and dependent on welfare.
The second pattern, which includes only three cases or
25% of the total number of subjects, contrasts sharply
with the first pattern; this second group is characterized by a late-born child of a married woman over 30
years of age. In the remaining three cases there is no
apparent association of variables.

Table V presents the chronological age of the child
at the time the study was completed and data on changes
in the marital status of the mother, mobility, and
changes in household composition. Some of the data on
this latter variable overlap with data in the two former
variables, as changes in marital status or mobility often
represent changes in household composition. The table
also includes reported evidence of psychiatric disorders
in the mother.

Case 03 is included in this table for the purposes
of identification; however, it is excluded from further
analysis because the pattern of disorganization in this
family was not captured by the present coding system.
This family was characterized by continuously shifting
household composition--the child's father, aunt, and the
mother's boyfriend lived there intermittently. Moreover,
although the mother had experienced no change in marital
status, both she and her boyfriend were free to engage
in simultaneous sexual relationships with additional
partners.

In addition to case 03, cases 05, 06, 09, and 11
present no changes in marital status throughout the
child's lifetime. Cases 05, 06, and 09 also show 0 or

TABLE IV. Relations Between Family's Source of Income, Maternal Age, Marital Status, and Child's Ordinal Position at Child's Birth

	50%									25%		
Welfare recipient	No	Yes	Yes	Yes	Yes	Yes	Yes	No	No	No	Yes	No
Maternal age	≤21	≤21	≤21	≤21	≤21	22	22	23	28	≥30	≥30	≥30
Marital status	S	S	S	S	S*	S*	M	M	M	M	M	M
Child's ordinal position	1	1	1	1	1	1	2	3	1A	≥4	≥4	≥4
Identification number	01	02	10	03	11	07	08	12	04	06	05	09

S* - Separated.
A - Adopted.

TABLE V. Significant Family Events during Child's Lifetime

Identification number	Age*	Changes in mother's marital status	Number of changes in address	Changes in household composition	Evidence of psychiatric disorder in mother
01	2 yr 6m	1. Single with boyfriend (father of child) 2. Single 3. Single with boyfriend-fiance 4. Married	4	1. Mo, child, mo's aunt and uncle 2. Mo, child, mo's girlfriend, girlfriend's mo and dtr 6. Mo, child, mo's husband (adoptive father)	None
02	4 yr 9m	1. Single with boyfriend (father of child) 2. Married to father of child 3. Separated for 6 mos. while husband in army	2	1. Mo, child, mo's mo 2. Mo, child, father 3. #2 and new sib	1. Suicidal ideation 2. Outpatient psychiatric treatment
03	1 yr 6m	No change; single with boyfriend (father of child)	1	1. Mo, child, boyfriend 2. Sister and sister's boyfriend sporadically	None
04	3 yr 8m	1. Married 2. Divorced 3. Divorced with boyfriend 4. Divorced	2	1. Foster family 2. Adoptive mo and father, child 5. Adoptive mo, child	None
05	4 yr 6m	No change; married	0	None	None
06	2 yr 3m	No change; married	1	None	None
07	3 yr 3m	1. Separated-divorced 2. Divorced with boyfriend 3. Married	1	1. Mo, child, mo's mo and bro 2. Mo, child, mo's husband (stepfa), step-bro 4. Mo, child, stepfa, half-sib	None

	Age*	Marital status	No.	Household composition	Psychiatric
08	4 yr 2m	1. Married 2. Divorced 3. Divorced with boyfriend 4. Common-law marriage	4	1. Mo, child, father, sib, fa's parents 2. Mo, child, fa, sib, mo's mo → 7. Mo, child, sib, half-sib, common-law husband (father of half-sib)	1. Attempted suicide 2. Outpatient psychiatric treatment
09	3 yr 10m	No change: married	0	None	1. Outpatient psychiatric treatment
10	3 yr 5m	1. Single 2. Single with boyfriend-fiance (not father of child) 3. Single 4. Single with boyfriend (not father of child) 5. Single	2	1. Mo, child, mo's parents 2. Mo, child → 4. Mo, child	None
11	1 yr 2m	None: divorced with common-law husband (father of child)	1	1. Mo, child, mo's fa 2. Mo, child, father (common-law husband)	None
12	2 yr 6m	1. Married 2. Separated- divorced 3. Divorced with boyfriend-fiance	2	1. Mo, child, father, sibs 2. Child, sibs, aunt, uncle, cousins → 5. Mo, child, sibs, mo's mo, boyfriend-fiance	1. Attempted suicide 2. Outpatient psychiatric and marital treatment 3. Psychiatric hospitalization

*Age of child at termination of study.

1 change of address and no changes in household composition. By contrast cases 01, 02, 04, 07, 08, 10, and 12
present one or more changes in marital status, residence,
and household composition.

To cluster the data on each of the variables just
discussed, the number of changes in household composition
and in the mother's marital status were both subdivided
into (1) no changes and (2) 1 or more changes. Evidence of
psychiatric disorder was categorized as present or
absent. Further, in order to avoid spurious relation
because number of changes in address or in marital status
is related to changes in household composition, mobility
was excluded from the analysis of clusters and only those
changes in household composition independent of change
in marital status were taken into account.

Table VI shows relations between variables and the
formation of two family patterns. First, families with
changes in household composition also had frequent changes
in marital status. By contrast, families without changes
in household composition had no changes in marital status.
In addition, there were more cases having evidence of
psychiatric disorders among the groups of families with
changes in the family unit. The question now raised is
how do these patterns relate to those observed at the
time the child was born.

Table VII shows the relationship between characteristics of the child's family at the time of the child's
birth and changes that have occurred during the child's
lifetime. The top row of 3 boxes represents the child's
family at the time of his birth. The bottom 2 boxes
represent events that occurred during the child's lifetime. The bar graphs within these 2 boxes indicate the
frequency with which the families experienced change in
household composition, changes in mother's marital status,
and evidence of psychiatric disorder in the mother.

As shown by the right side of the table, all three
families in Pattern 2--children born to older, married,
grandmultiparous women--experienced few or no changes
during the child's lifetime in the areas considered. By
contrast, as shown by the left side of the table, four
of the five families in Pattern 1--first-born children of
single women on welfare--had experienced many changes.
Only one case, 11, showed few changes. Furthermore, the
three families that did not conform to either Patterns 1

TABLE VI. Relations between Changes in Household Composition, Changes in Mother's Marital Status, and Evidence of Psychiatric Disorder in Mother during Child's Lifetime (N = 11)*

Identification number	08	01	02	07	02	04	10	11	05	06	09
Number of changes in household composition, independent of mother's marital status	4	4	2	2	1	1	1	–	–	–	–
Number of changes in mother's marital status	3	3	2	2	2	3	4	–	–	–	–
Evidence of psychiatric disorder	+	–	+	–	+	–	–	–	–	–	–

* Case 03 is omitted because the mother's marital changes are non-codable.

TABLE VII. Relations of Child's Ordinal Position, Mother's Marital Status, Age, and Family's Source of Subsistence with Significant Family Events during Child's Lifetime

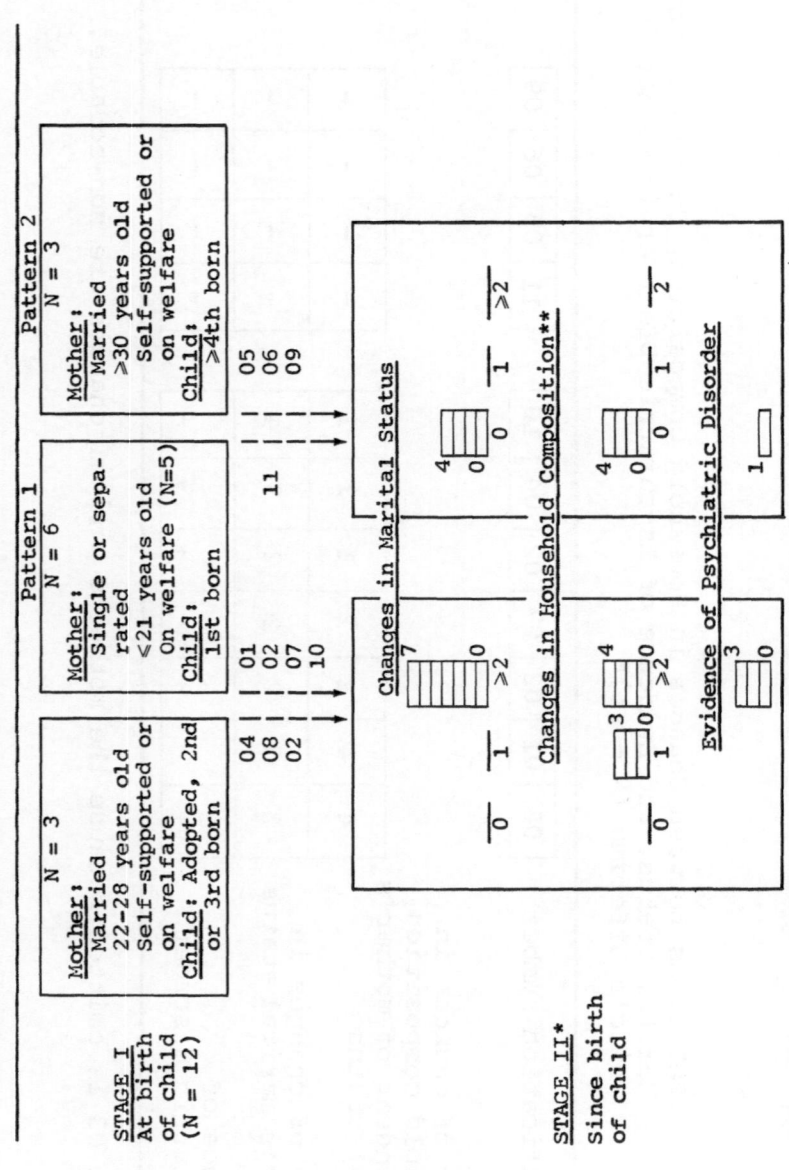

*Case 03 was omitted because the mother's marital changes are non-codable.
**Independent of changes in marital status.

or 2 at the time of the child's birth experienced many significant changes during the child's lifetime, thus making them similar to the Pattern 1 families at the termination of the study.

Data on the food purchasing practices of these families further illustrated the complexity of the problem and the difficulty of understanding why some of these children do not thrive. This aspect of the study included interviews regarding the type and frequency of foods purchased within 7 food groups: (1) vegetables, (2) fruits, (3) meats, fish, and poultry, (4) sugars and oils, (5) milk and milk products, (6) breads and cereals, and (7) snacks. For this presentation only the data on vegetables, fruits, and meats, fish, and poultry is discussed.

The food items purchased, for each of these three food groups, were analyzed using a Guttman scale. In this procedure items are ordered according to frequency purchased and cases ranked according to the number of items purchased. The coefficient of reproducibility, which indicates the degree to which the scale conforms to a perfect scale, is calculated from this ranking. The coefficients of reproducibility for vegetables, fruits, and for meats, fish and poultry are high. Thus a reader of the scale can predict quite accurately all items in a food group purchased by a family from the item purchased by the family which is least frequently bought by the group as a whole. Further, the nonparametric coefficient of concordance ($W = 0169$, $p < 0.02$) shows a similarity of rank orders and thus of variety purchased within each of the three food groups for each family.

This explanation on food purchasing practices serves the purpose of clarifying the behavior of the families presented in the table. The three large families where the mothers were 30 years old or older and where the child was late-born are among the five families with the highest degree of complexity in the diet (note here that we are discussing complexity, not volume). The question then is why the target children failed to thrive under such apparent optimal circumstances.

COMMENTS

The data presented stem from too few cases to warrant generalization. Still the data are of heuristic value and suggest that the development of preschool malnutrition

is likely to be associated with certain family characteristics. The strongest association we found was between
stunted growth in the child and a young unwed mother,
with frequent changes in marital relationship and domi-
cile. The vulnerability of low-income families with an
absent father is well documented in the literature and
should not be taken as surprising.

The second pattern we found--children born to older
married women of high parity from stable families--is
more surprising, especially because the data we have on
their food purchasing suggest adequacy of their diets.
The extent to which the large size of the family limits
availability of the diet to the child remains to be
studied.

Stunted growth without an organic cause and
associated with deficient nutritional intake in a
family whose income is high enough to warrant a
balanced diet is an indication of a failure in the
socialization process. In these cases it is apparent
that the transaction of the family with the child short-
changed the latter as he is deprived of the required
amount of nutrients--which are absolutely necessary for
his growth and preparation to become a productive
member of society. It is not difficult to imagine ways
in which a highly mobile family with frequent marital
change may fail to perceive the developmental needs of
a child. Finally, by placing the development of malnutrition within the theoretical framework of socialization and describing it as an inoperant transaction
between family and child, it becomes easy to recognize
the possibility that the psychological development of
these children is also affected by this failure of
socialization.

ACKNOWLEDGMENT

This work was supported by Contract (NIH) 73-447
with the National Institutes of Child Health and Human
Development.

LONGITUDINAL STUDY OF LANGUAGE DEVELOPMENT IN SEVERELY MALNOURISHED CHILDREN

Joaquín Cravioto and Elsa DeLicardie

Scientific Research Division

Hospital del Niño Iman, Mexico

At the community level, malnutrition—more specifically protein-calorie malnutrition—is a man-made disorder characteristic of the lower socioeconomic segments of society, particularly of the preindustrial societies, where the social system consciously or unconsciously creates malnourished individuals, generation after generation, through a series of social mechanisms among which limited access to goods and services, limited social mobility, and restricted experiential opportunities at crucial points in life play a major role.

When applied to an individual, the term protein-calorie malnutrition is a generic name used to group the whole range of mild to severe clinical and biochemical signs present in children as a consequence of a deficient intake and/or utilization of foods of animal origin, accompanied by variable intakes of rich carbohydrate foods. Kwashiorkor and marasmus are the names given in the Anglo-Saxon literature to the two extreme clinical varieties of the syndrome occurring in infants and children. The appearance of marasmus or kwashiorkor is related to the age of the child, the time of full weaning, the time of introduction of food supplements to breast milk, the caloric density and protein concentration of the supplements actually ingested by the child, and to the frequency and severity of infectious diseases present during weaning.

Recently research in the field of malnutrition has centered on the question of later functioning of individuals who suffered from the condition in early life. A series of studies done in various parts of the world has shown that survivors of early severe malnutrition differ from well nourished children in a great variety of functional aspects ranging from psychomotor behavior to intersensory organization (Cravioto et al., 1962, Pollitt et al., 1967, Chase et al., 1970, Bothe-Antoun et al., 1968, Yatkin et al., 1970, Liang et al., 1967, Monckeberg, 1968, Cravioto et al., 1966, Cravioto et al., 1971b, Cravioto et al., 1970, Cravioto et al., 1971a, Champakam et al., 1968). The problem at present is to separate the specific role that the deficient food intake may have from the contribution of other factors that interfere with the correct functioning of the individual. The reason for this rests in the fact that malnutrition in humans is an ecologic outcome (Cravioto, 1970), with many of the factors which either cause or accompany malnutrition being in themselves capable of influencing, in a negative way, mental and behavioral development. It is obvious that this type of research question can only be approached through the longitudinal observation of children at risk and with use of appropriate controls. With this idea in mind, since March 1966 we have been engaged in an ecologic study of a cohort of children born in a community where preschool malnutrition is highly prevalent, and where other factors related to the life of the children have variations of sufficient range to permit associative analyses to be carried out.

In brief, the project is the study of a total one-year cohort of children, all of them born in a rural village between March 1, 1966, and February 28, 1967. These children and their families have been closely observed from the nutritional, pediatric, socioeconomic, and developmental points of view in a coordinated manner, with great attention to detail, and so far as feasible using validated research instruments--a good number of them devised and tested by the project staff during the 10 years previous to the start of the induction of the cohort.

The objective of the study is to analyze the relationship between the conditions surrounding care of a child, especially those which correlate his nutrition to the course of his physical growth, mental development, and learning.

The main hypothesis to be tested is that intellectual growth at all stages and performance at school age will be related to the nutritional and health conditions to which the child has been exposed.

The children first brought into the study during the prenatal period have been followed for 5 years and will continue to be observed until they have completed 7 years of life (March, 1974); the earliest time at which certain crucial mental examinations can be meaningfully applied, and at which time the children can all be assessed in the relatively uniform environment of a primary school.

While the particular focus of the project is the relation between nutrition and mental development, by the nature of both variables the design is that of an ecologic study of young children in their family and social environments. The ecologic approach was selected on the basis that it constitutes a particular form of the natural history method which seeks to determine the nature of effective variables through a consideration of their interrelations in a single population. When applied to the problem of malnutrition, it attempts to identify patterns of cause and consequence by considering the interrelations among nutritional, health, and social factors. Moreover, by orienting itself longitudinally, the ecologic approach can identify age-specific conditions at risk, relate antecedents to consequences at different developmental stages, and integrate biological and social time scales. It can consider both the general and the microenvironment of the developing individual and deal with the interaction of biological and social variables. Perhaps most important for its usefulness is the fact that it incorporates uncontrolled variation as a fact of study. A basic requirement for the use of the ecologic method is, therefore, sufficient variation in the attributes to be considered in the population studied. If such variation is present, associative analysis can serve to identify, to segregate, and to interrelate the factors influential in affecting the consequences with which one is concerned.

Through the use of the ecologic method we plan to analyze:

a. The influence of social, economic, and familial circumstances on the development of malnutrition.

b. The effect of malnutrition on physical growth,
mental development, and learning.

c. The interaction of nutritional factors with
infectious disease, family circumstances, and social
circumstances on the processes of growth and development.

The intensive analysis to be done can be understood
only through a detailed acquaintance with the setting of
the study, the cohort under observation, and the measures
used.

THE SETTING OF THE STUDY

In order to examine the complex set of variables
with which our investigation is concerned, we have had to
study a large group of children. Estimates of sample
needs demanded the selection of a community of sufficient
size to provide at least 250 births in the annual cohort
to be followed longitudinally. The community selected
also had to contain a considerable range of social conditions and nutritional status as well as to be one in
which the population was likely to be cooperative and
willing to enroll and to remain in the study. Clearly,
for a longitudinal study, it was essential that the
population be relatively stable and that a high proportion of the families and infants enrolled for study at
birth be likely to continue to live in the community for
the duration of the period of inquiry.

The community chosen met these requirements:
Selection was based on previous experience with rural
communities and field studies. In one of these previous
studies the village chosen was a participating community
and had exhibited a high level of population stability
over time, excellent cooperation, and a wide range of
variation in social, economic, familial, and health
attributes. Furthermore, its annual birth expectancy
was 300.

The village is located in a semitropical subhumid
zone in southwestern Mexico in a primarily agricultural
region in which arid hillsides alternate with fertile
valleys and meadows. It is at an altitude of between
900 and 950 meters above sea level and has a hot sub-
tropical climate modified by its altitude. The median
annual temperature is between 23°C and 25°C in the
shade, and it ranges from chilly winters to very hot

summers in which daily high temperatures of 40°C are not uncommon. A small river whose waters are used both for irrigation and for laundering and other general purposes runs through the village.

As is characteristic of Mexican rural villages in this region, the arrangement of the town devolves from a central shaded plaza and proceeds centripetally along a series of unpaved and rutted dirt streets which are related to one another to form roughly quadrangular blocks. A street map of the village is presented in Figure 1. The small inclusion at the upper right of the figure indicates the arrangement of households within two specific blocks.

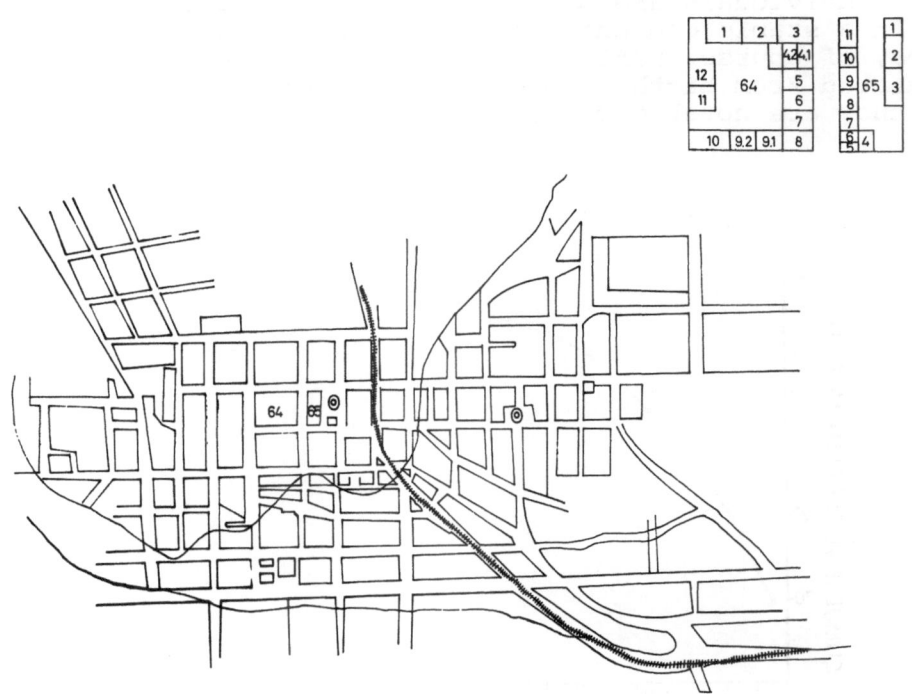

FIGURE 1. A street map of the village. The small insert at the upper right of the figure indicates the arrangement of households within two specific blocks.

The area surrounding the town site is entirely
agricultural, with sugar cane constituting the major
commercial crop. Small amounts of cotton and rice are
also grown commercially. Interspersed among the large
commercially organized fields are small family parcels
and rentable areas that are used by the villagers for
the production of food crops--principally corn, chilies,
tomatoes, and other garden crops and fruits for their
own consumption.

In 1965 we carried out a census of all village
households. Findings of the census indicated the presence of 5637 persons from 0 to 85 years of age organized in
1041 families. The numbers of men and women were in-
significantly different--2830 men and 2807 women. The
distribution by age and sex in the population are presented in Figures 2 and 3. As may be seen from both
figures, the population is relatively young; fully 50%
of the individuals are under 15 and 80% are under
35. In a stable community such as this one these age
ratios, of course, reflect a reduced life expectancy
calculated from birth. No differences in age-specific
frequency are notable by sex.

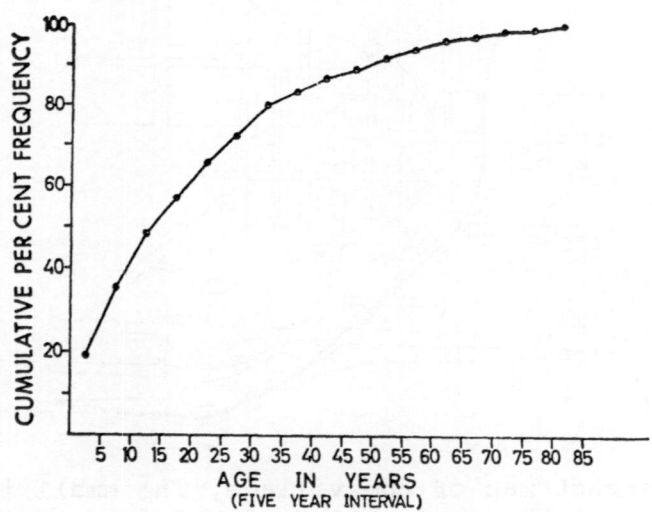

FIGURE 2. Distribution of population in the village by
          age.

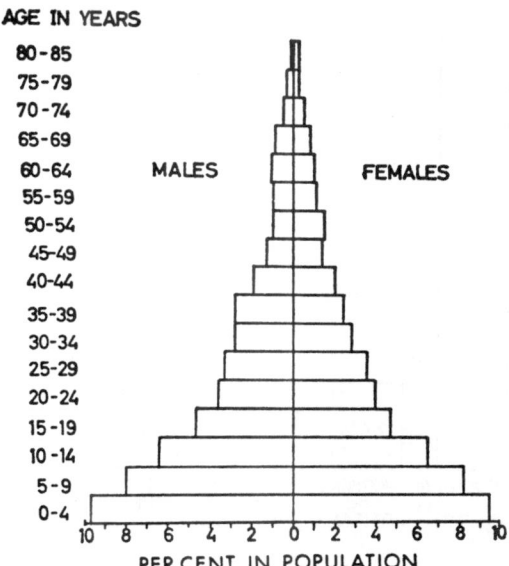

FIGURE 3. Age and sex of the village population.

Birth rates over the past 20 years had been at a mean value of approximately 55 per thousand and led to an annual expectancy of approximately 300. In the 12-month series of births upon which the current study is based, the predicted expectation was fulfilled.

The principal occupation of the villagers is agriculture, although relatively small numbers of people are employed as workers and artisans, and a still smaller number are engaged in commerce or in the practice of a profession. The occupations are reflected in terms of the main sources of family income as presented in Figure 4: approximately 65% of the population gains its livelihood directly from agriculture; 12.5% work at a variety of jobs, including transport workers, laborers in the small cotton gin or mattress factory, carpenters, masons, or other skilled and semiskilled crafts; and 9% are small tradesmen, shopkeepers, or teachers. Included in the last

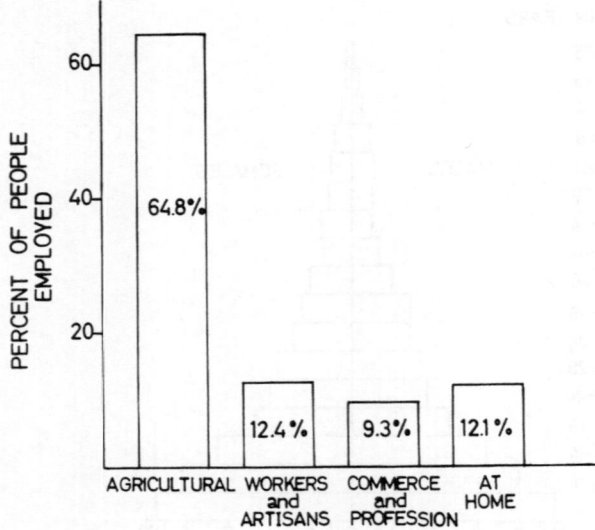

FIGURE 4. Main sources of family income in the village.

group are one architect, one engineer, and two physicians who served both the village proper and the surrounding communities.

The social and economic status of people who work
in agriculture is by no means homogeneous, as can be
seen in Figure 5. The preponderance of persons are
agricultural day laborers (jornaleros) whose employment
is seasonal and whose income is marginal. These workers
supplement their income by the seasonal planting of food
crops on communal lands at some distance from the village.
A second group comprising some 23% of those engaged in
agriculture have family plots that are cultivated both
for small-scale commerce and for self-use. The best
situated cultivators are either small owners or renters
of relatively high-grade farmlands; taken together,
these two groups constitute approximately 7% of those
engaged directly in agriculture as the main source of
family income.

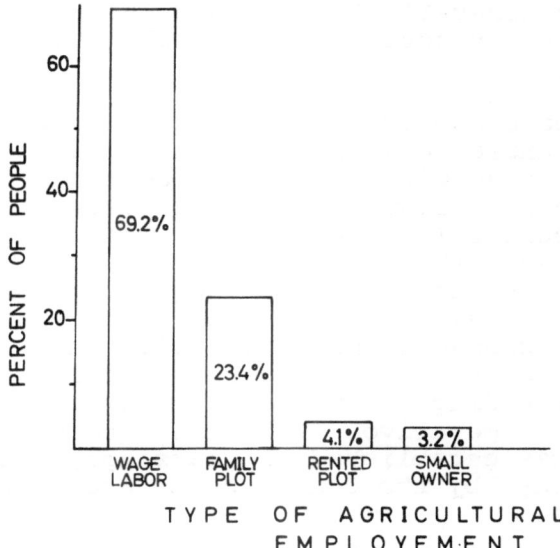

FIGURE 5. Proportions of people engaged in different
         types of agricultural work.

A few words are required to describe the different
types of landholding if the different relations to
agriculture are to be understood. The jornalero owns
no land and works entirely for wages. He is, in the
main, not insured for social and health services and
represents the most economically deprived and unstable
segment of the population. He can be described as an
agricultural proletarian.

The ownership of land by individuals is of two
kinds, the first of which is the family plot (ejido).
These are small parcels of land ranging generally from
one to three acres that were distributed to landless
peasants (peones) at the time of the agrarian reform.
Such land is held by the family in perpetuity so long
as it is worked, but it may not be sold, traded, divided,
or attached for debt. All of the ejidos owned by the
villagers have been amalgamated into a sugar cooperative.
The second type of individual land ownership is represented by the small proprietors whose plots are generally
larger than the ejidos. Their plots may be bartered,
sold, mortgaged, attached for debt as private property,

and divided or sold with no special limitations. The
rented lands are generally larger, and those who operate
them are economically better off than the other agricultural groups.

Until 30 years ago the village was almost totally
agricultural in character. Since then it has been in
a state of slow transition to a mixed economy representing more advanced levels of both industrial technology and agricultural organization. The beginning of
the transition was marked by a national law authorizing
and facilitating the development of agricultural com-
bines and cooperatives. Shortly after this law was
enacted, a large cane-growing cooperative and a sugar
refinery 17 km from the village were established. Much
of the land surrounding the village was assimilated
into this large cooperative. A mattress factory employing 20 workers was established 12 years ago, and this was
followed in 5 years by the construction and operation of a
small cotton gin.

These changes in economic base have been accompanied
by greater availability of transportation, the improvement and construction of roads, and a considerable increase in the amount of interaction between people in
the village, and more advanced urban and semiurban
centers. The technologic advances have been accompanied,
too, by the improvement of a variety of village services
including schools, a central water supply, and a social
welfare and health center. The village now has one
kindergarten, two primary schools, and one school accept-
ing pupils to the ninth grade. Attendance at school is
compulsory starting at 7 years of age and continuing for
6 years; beyond this, further study may be continued on an
elective basis for 3 years inside the village and for
higher levels of study outside it.

Variation in health conditions in the community and
in the relative opportunities available for the growth
and development of children are reflected in two sets of
data. The first of these deals with the weights and
heights of schoolchildren. A comparison of the growth
attainment of children attenting school in 1965 with the
growth of children who were at school a generation
earlier suggest that the technologic changes have not
been accompanied either by a change in mean height or
weight for age or by any diminution in the variability
of these characteristics in the population. The Wetzel
grids presented in Figure 6 illustrate this lack of
change.

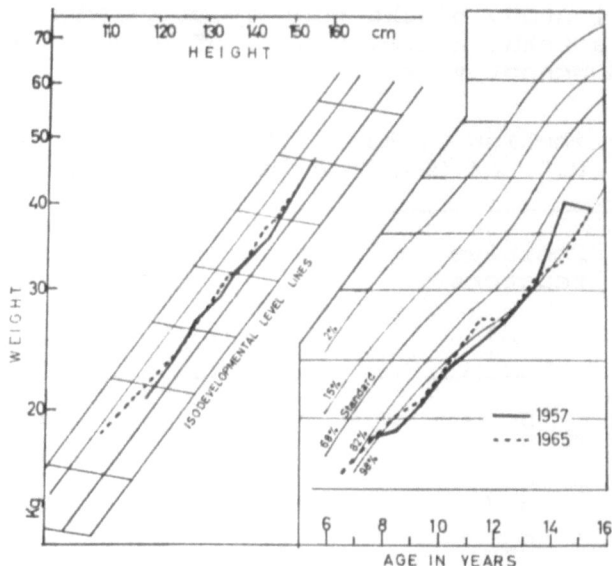

FIGURE 6. Comparative Wetzel Grids of height and
weight in two generations of schoolchildren.

The second set of data uses tuberculin reactivity
as an index of health risk and reflects a high frequency of the children's exposure to sources of infection, with age-specific values for positive reaction
to tuberculin showing a continuing rise of positive
reactors with age as can be seen in Table I.

As a final step in assessing the suitability of
the village for our purposes, a sampling survey was
made of households with children of preschool age for
clinical evaluation of children and the assessment of
the prevalence of subnutrition as indicated by a depression of height for age, as can be seen in Table II.

The figures indicate that at all age levels in
the preschool period, mild, moderate, and severe degrees
of malnutrition are present in the community with a
frequency that makes it a fair representative of communities in which chronic subnutrition is prevalent.
All of the data considered provided a basis for selecting the community as a suitable site in which to conduct

a longitudinal study of the ecology of growth and development in a total annual cohort of births over the
preschool and school years.

TABLE I. Distribution by Age of the Positive Reactors
         to P.P.D. of Children in the Village

Age (yr)	Positive reactors (%)	Age (yr)	Positive reactors (%)
3	0	11	12.3
4	0	12	12.6
5	3.7	13	16.1
6	2.1	14	15.9
7	7.8	15	20.0
8	12.4	16	37.5
		Total	10.8

TABLE II. Nutritional Status of Preschool Children in
          the Village

Age (months)	Number of children	Malnutrition (%) Third degree	Malnutrition (%) Mild-moderate	Normal (%)
0-5	132	0	5	95
6-11	112	3	9	88
12-23	210	5	18	77
24-35	207	9	21	70
36-47	212	8	8	84
48-59	201	5	11	84

THE BIRTH COHORT

The Children

Of the 300 infants born during the 12-month period
in which the cohort of births was collected, there were
equal numbers of boys and girls, with the social origins
of these children closely following the distribution of
principal sources of income and occupation in the
village as a whole. Minor differences from the overall distribution can be attributed wholly to the con-
striction in age range associated with reproduction.

The manner in which principal sources of family
income were represented in the cohort are presented in
Figure 7. The great majority of families were agricultural, with 66% of all children from such families.
Sixteen percent of the children were born to families
of workers and artisans, with four times as many of the
former type of family as of the latter represented.
Equal numbers of tradesmen and professional families
were present in the 4.5% of the births among these
social groups. Some 13% of the births occurred in
families in which it was difficult or impossible to define an intrafamilial source of income. These families
were ones in which the mother and children were mainly
dependent upon some other familial or social source of
support; they are labeled <u>at home</u> in Figure 7.

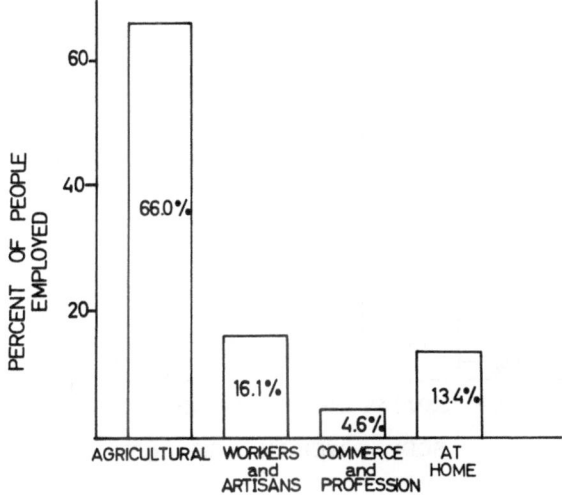

FIGURE 7. Main sources of family income in the cohort.

The distribution of birth weights in the annual
cohort is presented in Figure 8. There were eight infants weighing 1500-1999 g, twenty-eight weighing 2000-
2499 g, 147 weighing 2500-2999 g, 86 weighing 3000-3499
g, and 22 weighing 3500-3999 g. Mean birth weight was
2898 ± 444 g. A birth weight of less than 2500 g was
thus obtained for 12.3% of the cohort, whereas only 7.6%
of the children weighed more than 3500 g. As would have
been expected from other bodies of data, the mean birth
weight of boys was significantly higher than that of
girls (Figure 9). The mean birth weight of boys was
2977 ± 394 g, and that of girls 2860 ± 408 g. The mean
difference of 117 g was significant at the 0.02 level of
confidence.

The distribution of total body length at birth for
the children in the cohort is presented in Figure 10.
The median body length was 48.5 cm, with 25% of the
children having a body length of less than 47 cm and an
equal number of children having body lengths between 49.5
and 53 cm. As was the case for birth weight, mean body
length at birth was significantly higher in boys than
in girls. As may be seen from Figure 11, boys had a
mean length value of 48.7 ± 1.8 cm and girls one of
48.0 ± 2.0 cm. This difference, though small absolutely,
is statistically significant (t = 3.3; p < 0.1).

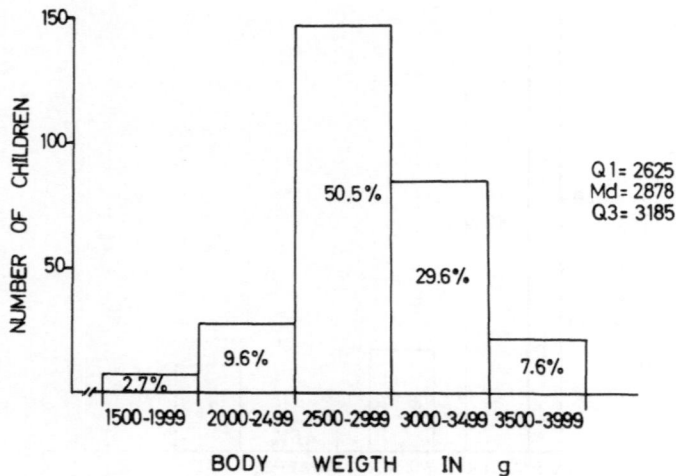

FIGURE 8. Birth weight of children in the annual cohort
        of births.

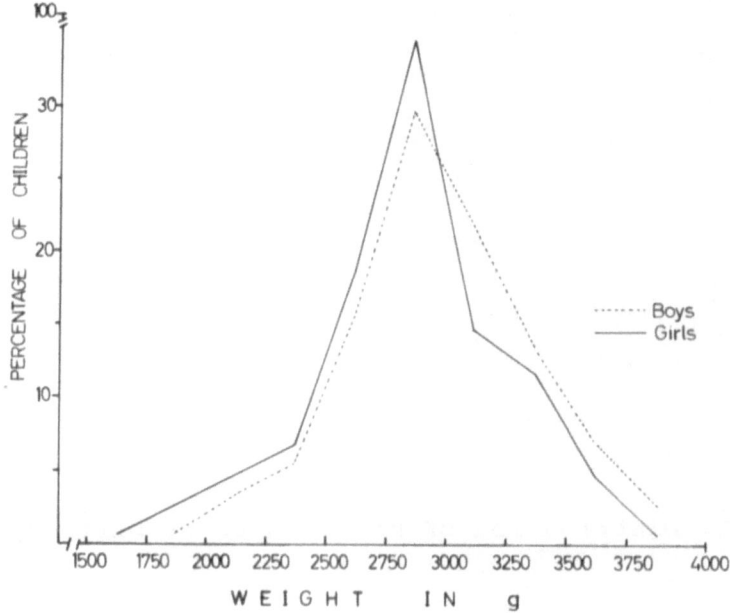

FIGURE 9. Distribution of body weight at birth by sex.

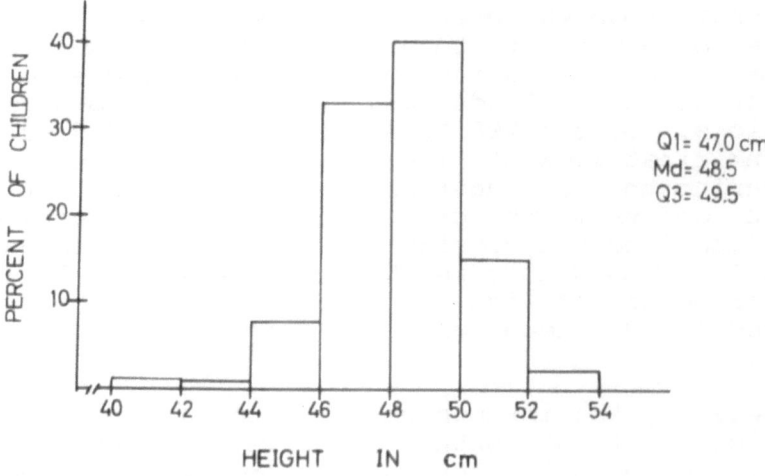

FIGURE 10. Distribution of total body length at birth
in cohort.

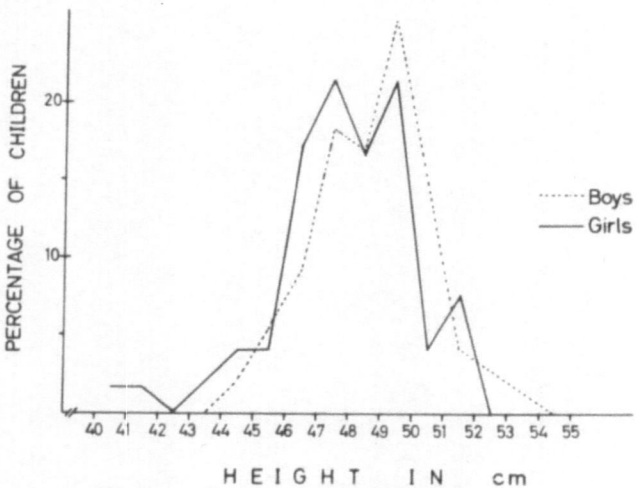

FIGURE 11. Distribution of body length at birth by sex.

Mortality and Emmigration

Of the 300 children delivered, 296 were alive at
birth and four were dead at delivery. No particular
occupational group was overrepresented in those stillborn: one child was born to a family whose principal
source of income was agricultural day-labor, one to a
cultivator of rented lands, and two others to owners of
family plots. Of the 296 live-born infants, 7 died
during the first week of life (23.6 per 1000) and 3
others during the remainder of the first month. If the
stillborns and those who died during the first week of
life are combined and considered as perinatal deaths,
the rate for such deaths is 36.7 per thousand. Com-
bining all deaths of live-born infants during the first
month results in a neonatal death rate of 33.8 per
thousand.

Generally, the infants who were stillborn or who
died during the first month of life were of low birth
weight. Unfortunately, through custom, those who were
stillborn or who had died a few hours after birth could not
be weighed. The remaining seven children had birth
weights below 2300 g.

Nine infants died during the remainder of the first year of life. Of these 7 died between the 2nd and 6th month of life. It is of interest that one of the two infants whose death occurred after 6 months of life was bitten mortally by a scorpion. These data taken as a whole indicate that 19 live-born infants in the cohort died in the first year of life with a resultant infant mortality rate of 63.3 per thousand.

The children who died were not randomly distributed in the cohort with respect to weight or body length at birth. With a mean birth weight in the cohort of 2898 g the mean weight at birth of the children who died during the first year of life was 2536 g. Similarly, mean body length of the deceased was 45.8 cm, as contrasted with a mean body length of almost 49 cm in the cohort as a whole. Both of these mean differences were significant at less than the 0.01 level of confidence. It was of course possible that these mean differences were contributed by an excess of premature infants in the infants who were stillborn or who died in the first year of life. Such a possibility is supported by the fact that six of the infants who died were premature. This number results in a prematurity of 260 per thousand deliveries which is more than twice the rate of 124 per thousand deliveries present or in the cohort as a whole. However, if one considers only infants above 2500 g at birth among the stillborn and infant deaths, one still notes a preponderance of poorly grown children with 63% of them having birth weights below the median of the cohort, and the remainder with weights only slightly higher than the median birth weight. Only 3 of the 23 infants had body lengths equal to or greater than the median of the cohort as a whole. Two of these were exactly at the median and one 1 cm higher; all other infants were between 1.5 and 7.0 cm shorter than the median body length for the whole cohort. It appeared therefore that those who were either stillborn or who had died during the first year of life were less well grown in utero than the survivors.

After the first year of life of the cohort 10 more children died. With the exception of two cases whose deaths were due to accidents (severe extensive burns, and bronchoaspiration) and a child who died of hypoprothrombinemia and purpura, all other deaths in this 4-year age period can be directly related to infectious disease accompanying severe malnutrition in most cases.

Table III shows the sex, age, and probable cause of each death occurring in the 0-5 yr period of study.

As may be derived from the cumulative frequency figures, all the children who left the program were at least examined during the newborn period. Forty-four out of the 50 children whose families emigrated from the village have data for the first 3 months of their life, 34 children completed 6 months of study. Twenty-two had at least one year of longitudinal observations, of these, 7 were seen for at least two years, and two children completed 3 years of longitudinal examinations. In all 50 cases family data are available.

TABLE III. Mortality in the Cohort During the First Five Years of Study

I. Stillborn

Number	Code	Sex	Age at death (days)	Cause of death
1	13.12	M	0	Unknown
2	13.5	F	0	Unknown
3	13.26	M	0	Unknown
4	4.22	F	0	Unknown

II. First Week of Life

1	12.24	F	1 hr	Unknown
2	13.28	F	1 hr	Unknown
3	7.12	F	5 hr	Bronchoaspiration
4	9.18	M	5 hr	Prematurity
5	6.11	M	6 hr	Hyaline membrane
6	8.24	M	2 d	Congenital malformation and bronchopneumonia
7	13.2	M	3 d	Bronchopneumonia

III. From 8 to 30 days

1	4.23	F	9	A.B.O. Incompatibility
2	2.3	F	17	Electrolyte disturbance
3	12.15	F	21	Prematurity

TABLE III. (Continued)

Number	Code	Sex	Age at death (days)	Cause of death
IV. From 30 to 360 days				
1	13.29	M	40	Electrolyte disturbance due to diarrhea
2	13.16	M	43	Pyelonephritis
3	12.14	F	76	Electrolyte disturbance due to diarrhea
4	10.13	F	78	Septicemia
5	11.2	F	85	Bronchopneumonia
6	11.27	F	130	Electrolyte disturbance due to diarrhea
7	12.17	F	139	Electrolyte disturbance due to diarrhea
8	7.11	F	268	Scorpion bite
9	5.24	M	312	Electrolyte disturbance due to diarrhea
V. From 1 to 5 years				
1	3.22	M	375	Severe electrolyte disturbance due to diarrhea
2	13.6	F	400	Bronchopneumonia, malnutrition
3	1.21	M	405	Bronchoaspiration
4	11.6	F	435	Bronchopneumonia, malnutrition
5	4.19	M	654	TB, miliar
6	2.22	F	737	Kwashiorkor amebiasis
7	11.20	M	1036	Kwashiorkor diarrhea
8	3.1	M	1229	Electrolyte disturbance due to diarrhea
9	9.13	M	1240	Third-degree burns
10	8.22	F	1413	Kwashiorkor purpura

TABLE IV. Time Spent in the Study by Children Who Left
the Program Because of Family Emigration

Days under observation	Number of children	Cumulative frequency
0	0	50
1-3	0	50
4-15	1	49
16-30	1	48
31-90	4	44
91-180	10	34
181-270	7	27
271-360	5	22
361-420	5	17
421-540	3	14
541-610	4	10
611-720	3	7
721-810	1	6
811-900	2	4
901-990	1	3
991-1080	1	2
1081-1170	0	2
1171-1260	1	1
1261-1350	0	1
1351-1440	1	0

Familial and Social Background

Broadly considered, background factors in the cohort
are of three kinds, relating, first, to the mother as a
biologic and social organism; second, to the family
structure; and third, to objective circumstances of life
such as sources of family income and housing conditions
for the family. Each factor will be considered in turn,
with the exception of sources of income, which have
already been presented.

We shall begin our consideration of the background
characteristics of the children by viewing some features
of the mother as a biologic organism--her age, height,
weight and previous pregnancies. The age distribution
of mothers in the cohort is presented in Figure 12. Age
ranged over 30 years; the mothers included two girls having
their first children at age 13, and one woman having a
child at 43. The mean age was 25.6 $\pm$ 6.8 yr, and the
median age was 24 yr, with 75% of mothers under 30 years of
age. The distribution of maternal age tends toward
bimodality and, as a whole, contains sufficient variability to permit associative analysis to be carried out.

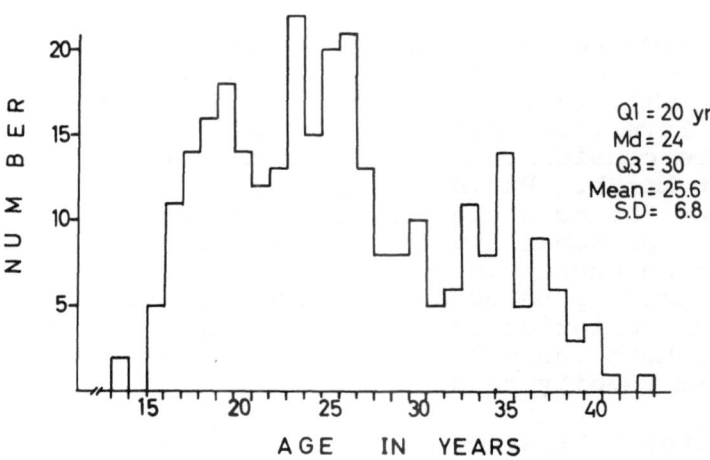

FIGURE 12. Age distribution of mothers in cohort.

The heights and weights of the mothers also varied widely (see Figures 13 and 14). The mother's heights ranged from 133 to 165 cm, with a mean value of 148.2 $\pm$ 2.8 cm. The heights are relatively normally distributed with a slight tendency for increased frequency in the lower range of stature. The median value was 147.5 cm, and 75% of the women were less than 153 cm tall.

Weight of the mothers ranged from 32 to 86 kg. This upper weight value was markedly atypical and is so indicated by a break in the distribution of values on the x axis of Figure 14. Mean weight was 53.0 $\pm$ 4.8 kg with a median value of 51 kg, suggesting a slight excess in frequencies at the lower end of the distribution. Both height and weight exhibit sufficient variability to make associative analysis feasible.

The distribution of pregnancy numbers in the cohort is presented in Figure 15. Pregnancy number ranged from one to more than 11, with the highest being 16. Relatively equal numbers of births occurred at pregnancy numbers 1-4. Higher pregnancy numbers in the cohort tended to occur with diminishing frequency. From the viewpoint of epidemiologic evidence in obstetrics, it is not meaningful to consider the distribution of parities in terms of mean value. Available evidence suggests that special conditions of risk attend first births and births which occur after the fifth pregnancy; enough cases in each of these parity ranges exist to permit analysis within the cohort of births.

In addition to the foregoing biological characteristics of the mothers, at least three other characteristics--the mothers' personal hygiene, literacy, and educational level, and contact with mass information media--can be considered in relation to the child's condition at birth. Ratings of personal hygiene ranged from a low of 20% to a high of 100%; the distribution of scores for personal hygiene are presented in Figure 16. The median score was 56.6%, with three fourths of the mothers scoring below an estimated cleanliness level of 76%. Wide variation in personal cleanliness existed among the mothers and subgroups differing in personal hygiene could readily be defined.

The mothers' literacy and school attainments are presented in Figure 17. Almost half the mothers were completely illiterate. Another 10% either had become literate from exposure to adult literacy campaigns or

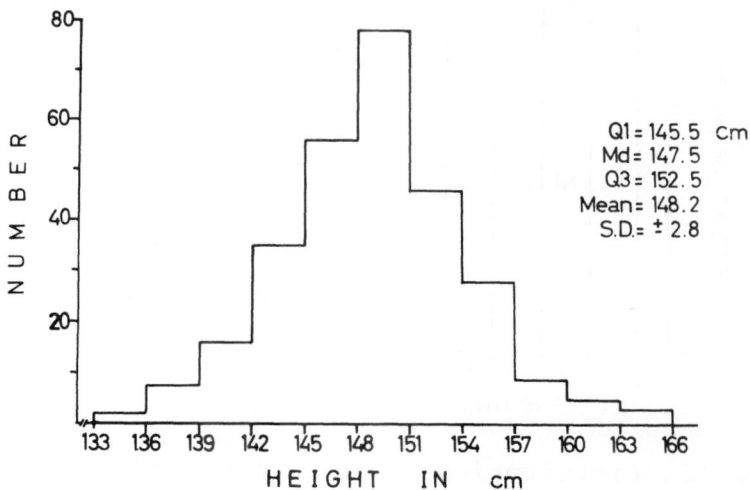

FIGURE 13. Height distribution of mothers in cohort.

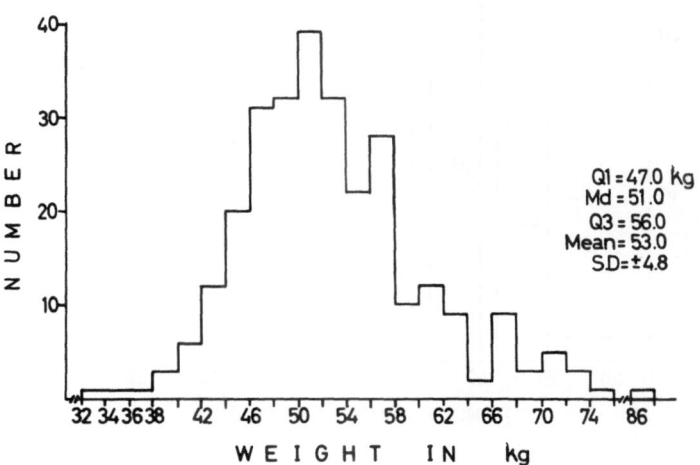

FIGURE 14. Weight of mothers in cohort.

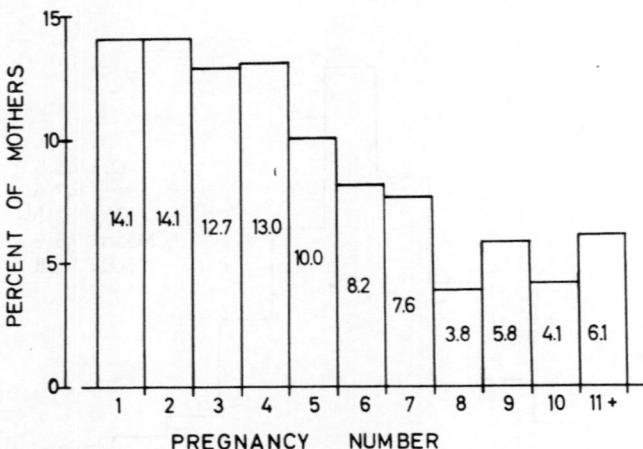

FIGURE 15. Distribution of pregnancy numbers in the cohort.

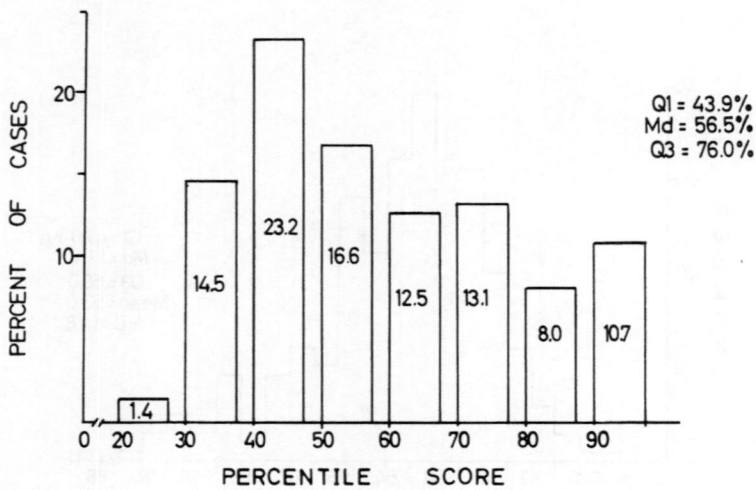

FIGURE 16. Personal hygiene of mothers in cohort.

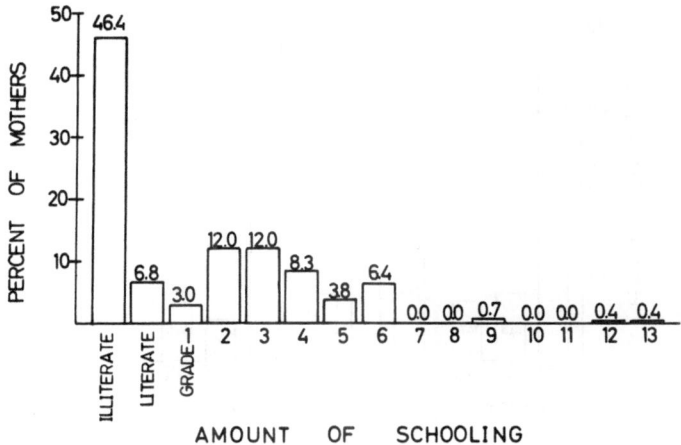

FIGURE 17. Literacy and school grade completed by
mothers in cohort.

had acquired basic literacy by the completion of one
school grade. Only 6.4% had completed the full primary
school curriculum of 6 yr, and a remaining 1.5% had
schooling beyond primary school. From a functional
point of view it was possible to group the mothers into
four classes: (1) the illiterates, (2) the adult
literates and those who had completed the first and
second grades, (3) those who completed the third
through the fifth grades, and (4) those who had completed primary school. These functional groupings have
been used in later associative analyses.

As may be seen from Figure 18 very few of the women
had any exposure to television. Half had little or no
regular contact with the radio, and almost 70% engaged
in no newspaper reading except episodically. If a consideration of newspaper reading is limited only to that
segment of the population that is literate, slightly
fewer than 50% of the mothers who were capable of reading newspapers actually did so. Thus, in the present
study we have viewed radio as the most effective medium
of disseminating mass information and have restricted
our consideration of the relation between the child's
characteristics and the mother's contact with mass media
to this medium.

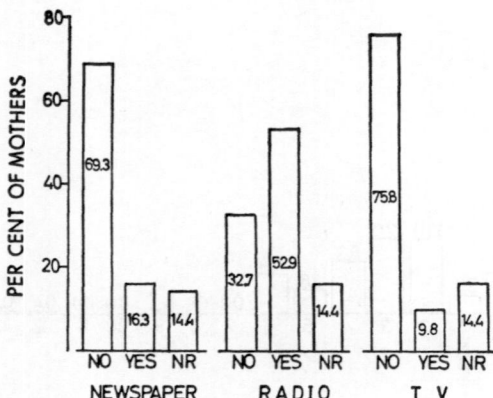

FIGURE 18. Contact of the mothers with mass information
          media.

Size and family and the sanitary structure of the
household, respectively, are presented in Figures 19
and 20. There is considerable variation for both of
these: family size ranges from a single-child family
of three individuals to both nuclear and extended
families of a dozen or more members.

The sanitary structure of the household also had
a wide range. Most households were substandard, but a
considerable number exhibited good to excellent conditions and facilities. Sufficient variation existed
to permit the sanitary structure of the household to be
related, as a differential background factor, to the
characteristics of the child.

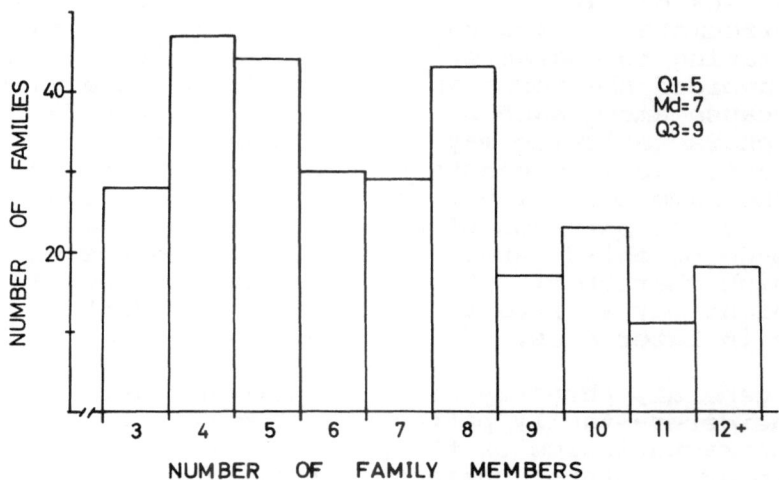

FIGURE 19. Size of the families in the cohort.

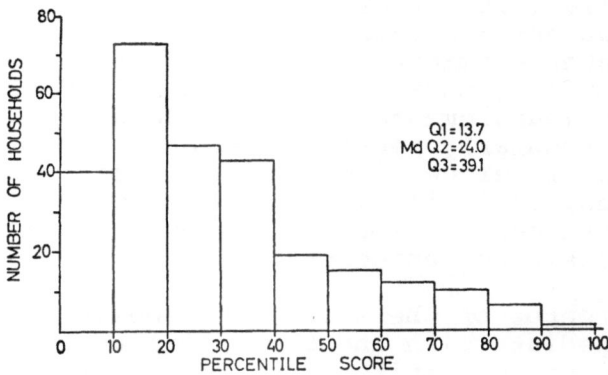

FIGURE 20. Objective conditions for sanitation in the
households in which the children lived.

THE VARIABLES

In the course of the study we have been concerned
with two sets of variables: those relating to the child's
family circumstances and background environment, and
those relating to characteristics of the child himself.
We have avoided the terms antecedent and outcome variables because among each of the general sets of factors
certain characteristics may be considered with equal
justification as antecedents or consequences of others
within the same set. Thus, the mother's education may
well affect her patterns of personal hygiene and pre-
ferred mode of child care. Similarly, among the variables which characterize the child, a factor such as
birth weight may well be an important antecedent for
outcomes in later ages.

In general, three types of background factors have
been considered--family pattern, biological and psychosocial characteristics of the parents and caretakers,
and macroenvironmental characteristics of the child
ranging from survival to evaluation of physical and
behavioral changes with age.

Data upon the basis of which ratings of the variables could be made were obtained by interview, by
direct observation and measurement, by assessments using
clinical methods, and by the application of special tests.

The reliability of all measures and ratings has been
assessed, and any measures with excessive levels of
intra- or inter-examiner, or score-rescore error were
either improved by modification or eliminated. For
somatometric measurements including weight and height,
scales were regularly recalibrated and examined. Errors
beyond the 2% level were considered excessive. For
rating scales, reliability levels expressed as retest
and/or rescore correlation coefficients of less than
0.82 were considered unacceptable.

The director of the study, the senior psychologist,
the senior pediatrician and the social worker-nutrition-
ist, as a research committee, shared the responsibilities
of quality control and maintenance of strict standardi-
zation and completeness in data collection. The senior
biostatistician of the project was a member of this
committee since the time he joined the team.

On each one of the 229 children remaining in the cohort at 5 years of age (300 births plus 12 arrivals during the first year of study, minus 33 deaths and 50 emigrations) the information outlined in Table V was obtained.

TABLE V. Data Collected on Each Child Studied

Variable	Measurement	Age period (yr)	Frequency
I. Growth			
a. Physical			
	Body weight	0-5	Bimonthly
	Height, chest and arm circumference	0-3	Monthly
		3-4	Bimonthly
		4-5	3/yr
	Skin-fold thickness	0-3	Monthly
		3-4	Bimonthly
		4-5	3/yr
	Bone age	4-5	1/yr
b. Mental			
	Psychomotor, adaptive, language and socialpersonal dedelopment	0-2	Monthly
		2-3	Trimestral
		3-4	3/yr
	Bipolar concept formation	2-3	3/yr
		3-4	2/yr
		4-5	2/yr
	Finger-thumb opposition	3-5	2/yr
	Finger localization	4-5	2/yr
	Wechsler preschool and primary scale of intelligence	4-5	2/yr
	Styles of response to cognitive demands	4-5	2/yr

TABLE V. (Continued)

Variable	Measurement	Age period (yr)	Frequency
	Sensory-motor and movement skills: static balance, dynamic balance visual-motor coordination involving aiming and accuracy, motor control and inhibition	4-5	2/yr

As the cohort is reaching the 5 to 6 year period the following tests are being added:

	Measurement	Age period (yr)	Frequency
	Spontaneous language	5-7	2/yr
	Psycholinguistic abilities: Language decoding (meaning) Language encoding (expression) Grammatical levels of decoding and encoding Development and growth of grammatical language	5-7	2/yr
	Visual perception Form recognition	5-7	2/yr
	Intersensory integration Visual-haptic Visual-kinesthetic Kinesthetic-haptic Auditory-visual	5-7 6-7	2/yr 2/yr
	Analysis and synthesis of geometric forms	6-7	2/yr
	Learning strategies	6-7	1/yr
	Concrete operations (Piaget)	6-7	1/yr

II. Nutrition

	Measurement	Age period (yr)	Frequency
	Food consumption (child)	0-2 2-3 3-4 4-5	Monthly Trimestral 2/yr 1/yr

TABLE V. (Continued)

Variable	Measurement	Age period (yr)	Frequency
	Familial food consumption	3-4 4-5	2/yr 1/yr
	Clinical signs of child's malnutrition	0-5	Bimonthly
III. Health			
	Prenatal and delivery history		Once
	Pediatric examination Morbidity history of child and of each member of the household	0-5	Bimonthly
IV. Mother-child interaction			
	Time-sample observation and inventory of home stimulation	0-3 0-3 3-4 4-5	Monthly Trimestral 2/yr 1/yr
V. Socio-cultural a. Familial			
	Family composition and organization Family type Family size	0-5	Once
	Main source of income and annual income	0-5	Once
	Sanitary facilities, Social morbidity, Social change, Informal net of communication and mortality record	0-5	Bimonthly
b. Parental (mother only) Biological			
	Age, weight, height	0-5	Once

TABLE V. (Continued)

Variable	Measurement	Age period (yr)	Frequency
	Parity and reproductive history	0-5	1/yr
Socio-cultural			
	Personal cleanliness	0-3 3-5	Monthly 3/yr
	Formal education and contact with mass media	0-5	1/yr
	Nutritional knowledge Health education Proclivity toward change and cultural mobility	0-5	Once
	Psychological profile Maternal attitudes, and intelligence performance	0-5	Once

LANGUAGE DEVELOPMENT AND MALNUTRITION

Having described in detail the setting of the study and the birth cohort we would like on this occasion to present the preliminary results of the study of certain language features in a group of children who developed clinical severe malnutrition.

During the first 5 years of life of the cohort, 22 children, 14 girls and 8 boys, were diagnosed as suffering from clinical severe malnutrition. It must be said that these cases appeared in spite of all medical efforts to prevent them. Age at the time of diagnosis ranged from 4 to 53 months, with a single case below 1 year of age, 9 children between 1 and 2 years, 8 cases between 2 and 3 years of age, 3 children with ages between 3 and 4 years, and one case diagnosed at 53 months of age.

Fifteen of the 22 cases corresponded to the clinical picture of kwashiorkor, the other seven cases were of the marasmic variety (Autret and Behar, 1954). The proportion of marasmus in females and males was 4:3, while the number of females with kwashiorkor was twice the number for boys. Due to the small number of cases these differences do not reach statistical significance.

Ten children, 6 with kwashiorkor and 4 with marasmus, were treated at home while 9 children with kwashiorkor and 3 with marasmus were treated in the hospital. Average duration of hospital stay was 30 days; none of the children stayed in the hospital for more than 60 days. No deaths occurred in the hospital-treated group. In contrast, 3 of the 10 children treated at home died. Of these two were of the kwashiorkor and one of the marasmic clinical type; their respective ages at the time of diagnoses were 12, 14, and 22 months. In all three patients death occurred within a period of 15 to 60 days after diagnosis. Of the 19 survivors one child emigrated from the village after his discharge from the hospital leaving a total of 18 cases under study.

In the present report, language development obtained in the 19 children who developed clinical severe mal-nutrition before the age of 39 months has been compared with the language development shown by a group of children of the same birth cohort who were never considered as severely malnourished, and who were matched at birth for gestational age, body weight and total body length.

As may be seen in Table VI and Figure 21, mean language development, as measured by the Gesell method (Gesell and Amatruda, 1951), is very similar in index cases and controls during the first year of life when only one case of severe malnutrition had been diagnosed. As time elapsed and more children became ill with severe malnutrition, a difference in language performance favorable to the matched controls became evident. The difference was more pronounced at each successive age tested.

Not only were mean values significantly lower in the index cases, the distribution of individual scores was also markedly different from that obtained in the control group. Thus for example, at 3 years of age (Figure 22) 11 children of the control group had language scores above 1021 days-equivalent and only one child scored below 720 days. As a contrast, while none of the children with past malnutrition scored above 960 days-equivalent, 12 cases had values below 720 days, with 3 of these children having language performances 6 months below that shown by the control children with the lowest scores.

TABLE VI. Language Development Scores Found in Severely Malnourished Children and Matched Controls (Days-Equivalent)

Age (days)	Birth	180	360	540	720	900	1080
Past or present Severe malnutrition	27±3.2	167±14.4	289±47.2	385±86.0	467±102.7	534±103.0	657±119.5
Controls	28±1	177±21.2	334±55.4	490±73.3	633±93.4	785±143.1	947±135.2
"t" test	1.37	1.69	2.69*	3.90*	4.80*	5.80*	6.53*

*Significant at less than 0.01.

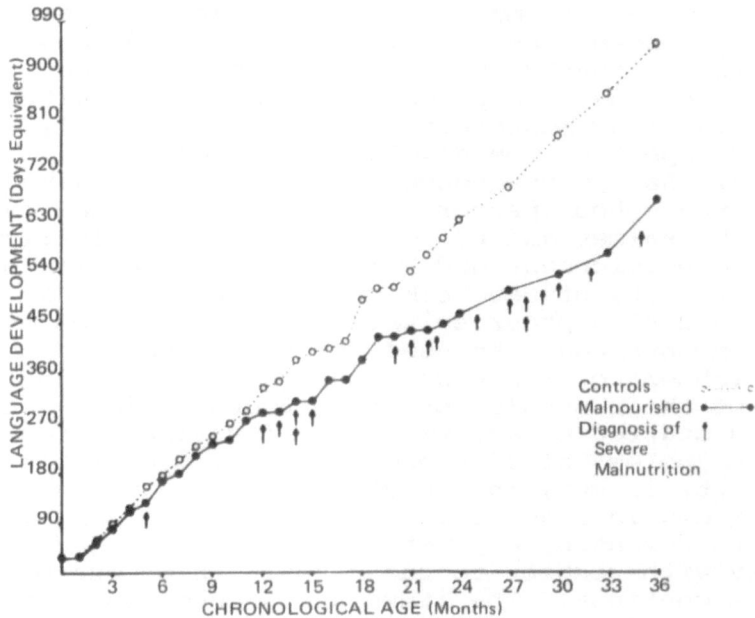

FIGURE 21. Mean language development as a function of
age in severely malnourished children and
matched controls.

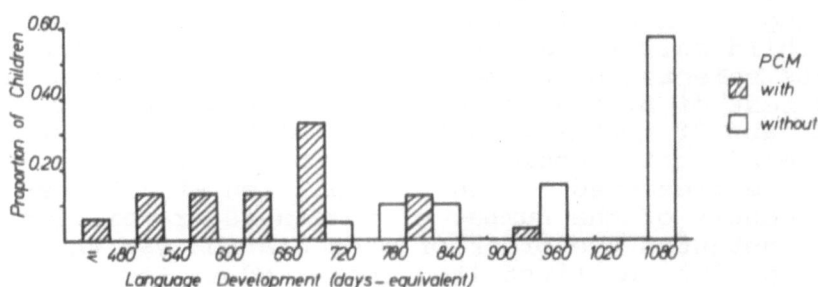

FIGURE 22. Proportion of children with or without PCM
with different language development score
at 1080 days of life.

Concept development and particularly the emergence
of verbal conceptions have long been viewed as a basic
factor in the development of human intelligence. The
emergence of the conception of opposites and with it
bipolar labeling represents an early and readily
measured aspect of the development of concepts in young
children. As a consequence of their concern with im-
proving the school performance of disadvantaged children,
Francis H. Palmer and his colleagues at the Institute
for Child Development and Experimental Education of the
City University of New York came to the view that the
development of a progressively difficult series of bipolar concepts could be used for the systematic training
and enrichment of language experience. Accordingly, as
a part of their studies on the effects of intervention
programs started at age two, they developed a test covering both "poles" of 23 concepts (e.g., big-little,
long-short, in-out) in two different situations. Most
of the items included require the child to select an
object representing a given pole from two objects differing only with respect to their position on one of the
concepts continua. The items are grouped into two forms
so that each form contains items covering both poles of
each concept. The forms differ only with respect to the
setting in which the concepts are placed. The score derived from the test provides a measure of the child's
knowledge of various categories that are commonly used
in organizing sensory experience.

Although Palmer and his associates have not viewed
the series of bipolar concepts that were developed to be
a language test, it is implicit in their protocols that
the progressively difficult training series could indeed
be used in itself, without training, as a measure for
assessing the natural acquisition of bipolar concepts in
young children. To test this hypothesis, 22 of the 23
concepts selected by Palmer were administered as a repeated test of bipolar concept acquisition at ages 26,
31, 34, and 38 months to a total cohort of children living
in a preindustrial society (Cravioto et al., 1969). All
items were presented to the 229 children at all ages
independently of the number of successes or failures.
In all instances the order of presentation was the same
beginning with the first item contained in Form I. Data
obtained at the successive ages tested clearly demonstrated a developmental course of competence in response
to tasks involving the utilization of bipolar concepts.

The competence in bipolar concept acquisition in children with past or present severe malnutrition and matched controls at successive ages is presented in Table VII and illustrated in Figure 23. As may be seen, the mean number of bipolar concepts present in the index cases in significantly lower that the mean number of concepts shown by the control group. It is important to remember that after 40 months all the children included in the malnourished group actually represent cases rehabilitated from clinical severe malnutrition, i.e., survivors considered as cured from the disease. It may be noted in this respect that the mean value found in the index cases at 46 months of age is almost twice the value obtained at 38 months. Nonetheless, the increment is not enough to bring the index cases to the value shown by the controls. In other words, the lag in language development found in severely malnourished children continued to be present after clinical recovery had taken place.

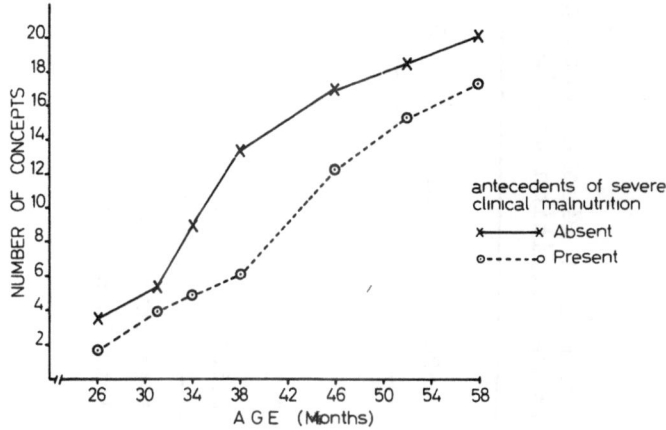

FIGURE 23. Number of bipolar language concepts present in children with and without antecedents of clinical severe malnutrition (Land of the White Dust).

TABLE VII. Mean Number of Bipolar Concepts Present in Children with Past or Present Severe Malnutrition and in Matched Controls

Age (months)	26	31	34	38	46	52	58
Past or present malnutrition	1.61±1.26	3.92±2.56	4.85±3.15	6.07±2.94	12.16±4.13	15.35±3.05	17.21±2.60
Controls	3.54±2.11	5.46±2.96	8.92±3.26	13.42±3.56	16.92±3.26	18.42±3.29	20.07±1.38
"d" Test	2.68*	1.42	3.36**	5.97**	3.23**	2.57*	3.66**

*Significant at less than 0.05.
**Significant at less than 0.01.

It has been repeatedly stated that human malnutrition does not occur in a vacuum, rather malnutrition is the outcome of an ecological situation characteristic of preindustrial societies (Cravioto et al., 1967). In the presence of a phenomenon with multiple causation, before interpreting our findings as due to the antecedent of severe malnutrition, it is necessary to try to sort out what other factors beside nutritional deficiency may be operating to interfere with the normal development of these children. Trying to answer this question we have compared the macroenvironment and some features of the microenvironment of the families of the severely malnourished children and of the matched control group.

Broadly considered, the macroenvironmental factors are of three kinds, relating, first, to the parents as biologic and social organisms; second, to the family structure; and third, to objective circumstances of life such as sources of family income, income per capita, and sanitary facilities present in the household. Since a detailed description of these factors has already been presented we will consider now the association of each one with the presence or absence of severe malnutrition.

Biological Characteristics of the Parents

Tables VIII and IX show the mean values for the biological characteristics of fathers and mothers. As may be seen, age, height, and weight of neither parent could discriminate between families with or without severely malnourished children. The number of pregnancies and the number of live children in the family also failed to separate families of malnourished children from families of the matched controls.

Sociocultural Characteristics

Personal cleanliness, literacy and educational level, and contact with mass information media were considered in relation to presence or absence of severe clinical malnutrition. The mean scores for personal cleanliness of the mothers of the malnourished and control groups were respectively 61 ± 20 and 68 ± 19. For the fathers the corresponding mean scores were 62 ± 16 and 61 ± 19. The differences in both sets fail to reach a level of significance of 0.05. Table X presents the distribution of literacy and formal educational level of

TABLE VIII. Mean Values for Certain Characteristics of
            the Fathers of Severely Malnourished
            Children and Matched Controls

	Severely malnourished children	Matched controls	"d"	p
Age (yr)	29.36+6.16	33.61+8.98	1.67	0.05
Height (cm)	159+7.2	162.5+5.88	1.58	0.05
Weight (kg)	57+7.36	60+10.7	0.99	0.05

TABLE IX. Mean Values for Certain Maternal Characteristics
          of Severely Malnourished Children and Matched
          Controls

	Severely malnourished children	Matched controls	"d"	p
Age (yr)	24.15+5.53	28.0+8.20	1.72	0.05
Height (cm)	148.0+6.42	149.5+6.82	0.70	0.05
Weight (kg)	49.6+5.04	52.7+7.23	1.50	0.05
Personal	60.6+19.9	67.6+19.3	1.07	0.05

TABLE X. Mother's Formal Education

School grade	Severely malnourished children	Matched controls	Total
Illiterates	2	3	5
Literates, 1st and 2nd grade	10	6	16
3rd grade	7	10	17
Total	19	19	38

Df = 2; x^2 = 1.72; "C" = 0.20.

the mothers. As may be seen there were 2 illiterate
mothers in the malnourished group, and 3 illiterate
mothers in the matched control group. A chi square
test shows that the differences in frequency distribution
of educational level are not significant ($p < 0.20$). Data
regarding father's literacy and educational level were
similar. Education change from maternal grandmother to
mother was estimated in both groups of children. Mean
change, i.e., number of grades gained or lost, was
1.07 ± 1.8, and 1.50 ± 3.3 in the malnourished and the control groups, respectively. The difference is not significant at the 0.05 level of confidence.

Contact with mass information media was explored
through reading of newspaper in literate parents and
radio listening. The number of mothers or fathers of
malnourished children who were regular newspaper readers
was not different from the number who did so in the
matched control group. Similarly, the number of fathers
who listened regularly to the radio was the same in both
malnourished and control groups. As may be seen in
Table XI, the case for the mothers was different. There
were almost equal numbers of radio listeners and nonlisteners in the malnourished group while the number of
listeners in the matched controls was more than 3 times
the number of nonlisteners. The difference is significant
at the 0.05 level of statistical confidence (chi square =
4.20; Df = 1; $p < 0.05$).

TABLE XI. Radio Listening by Mothers of Severely
Malnourished Children and Matched Controls

Mothers of	Radio listening		
	Yes	No	Total
Severely malnourished children	8	10	18
Matched controls	14	4	18
Total	22	14	36

X^2 = 4.20; Df = 1; p < 0.05.

Family Structure

Family size was not different in the malnourished
and the control groups. The number of members in the
families having a severely malnourished child was 7.4 $\pm$ 3.
This number is not statistically different from 7.2 $\pm$ 2.8
obtained for the families of the matched controls.

The frequency with which children belonged to extended or nuclear families was practically the same for
the malnourished and the matched control groups. Three
severely malnourished children were found in extended
families and 16 in nuclear families. The corresponding
figures for the matched controls were 4 in extended
families and 15 in nuclear families.

Family Economic Status

The socioeconomic status of the families was estimated using four indicators: main source of family income,
sanitary facilities present in the household, annual income per capita, and percentage of total expenditures
spent on food.

There was no difference in main sources of income
among the families of the malnourished and the control
children. Thirteen families in each group derived their

income from agricultural work, 12 as day-laborers and one
as a land-renter. The fathers of the other 6 families in
the control group were either workers or artisans. Among
the malnourished group 4 fathers were workers or artisans,
one was a small business owner, and one a public account-
ant.

Sanitary facilities of the households were substandard in both the malnourished and the control groups.
The percentage scores based upon the objective assessment of conditions and facilities for sanitation were
28 ± 17 for the homes of the malnourished children, and
31 ± 20 for the homes of the control children.

Although there was a tendency for the families of
control children to have a slightly higher annual per
capita income than families of severely malnourished
children, the difference was not large enough to become
significant even at the 0.10 level of confidence. Mean
annual income per capita, expressed in U.S. currency,
was 143 ± 78 dollars for the malnourished group and 168 ±
73 dollars for the control group.

The percentage of total expenditures spent on food
has long being considered a good indicator of level of
living. The greater the percentage spent on food the less
the purchasing power left for all other necessary expenditures (clothing, housing, education, religion, health,
etc.) and consequently the lower the economic condition
of the family. With these ideas in mind the percentage
of expenditures devoted to food procurement was calculated
on a yearly basis for the families of the malnourished
children and the controls. Mean percentage spent on food
was practically the same in both sets of families,
45.7% ± 15.2 for those families with severely malnourished
children, and 44.3% ± 16.3 for families of the control
children. The difference between groups is not statistically different at the 0.10 level of confidence.

In summary, of all the features of the macroenvironment considered, the only differential between severely
malnourished children and controls, matched at birth for
gestational age, body weight and total body length, was
the contact of the mother with the world outside the
village through regular radio listening. None of the
other characteristics of the parents (biological, social,
or cultural) or familial circumstances, including income
per capita, main source of income and family size, were
significantly associated with the presence or absence of
severely malnourished children.

Since the features of the macroenvironment could
not explain severe malnutrition, our attention has turned
toward the analysis of the microenvironments of the two
sets of children. We have selected the potential stimulation of the home as our first general indicator of the
quality of child care, and of the mother as the principal
stimulating agent in young children.

The instrument used for estimating home stimulation
was the inventory developed by Beattye Caldwell (1967).
This inventory was designed to sample certain aspects of
the quantity and, in some ways, the quality of social,
emotional, and cognitive stimulation available to a young
child within his home. Two forms of the inventory were
used, one designed for infants up to 3 years of age, and
the other one for children 3-6 years old. In both versions
the selection of items included has been guided by a set
of assumptions about conditions that foster development.
Accordingly, the inventory describes and quantitates
eight areas of the home environment: (1) frequency and
stability of adult contact, (2) vocal stimulation, (3)
need gratification, (4) emotional climate, (5) avoidance
of restriction, (6) breadth of experience, (7) aspects
of the physical environment, and (8) available play
materials. In each of these areas almost all items receive binary scores and no attempt is made to rate finer
gradations. The total score is the number of items recorded as positive for the child's development. If it
is desirable each area can be scored separately and related to specific features of development.

A trained psychologist scored the inventory of home
stimulation in every child in the cohort at six-month intervals during the first three years of life and at yearly
intervals thereafter. At the time of data collection and
of scoring the instrument, the psychologist was unaware
of the nutritional antecedents of the children.

Figures 24 and 25 show the distribution of home
stimulation total scores obtained in malnourished and
control children at 6 and 48 months of age. As may be
noted, even at 6 months, when only one case of clinical
severe malnutrition was present, the control children
had significantly higher home stimulation scores. Thus,
while none of these children had homes with less than 30
points, almost 25% of the homes of the future malnourished
children scored below 30, and almost 50% had scores below
32 points. Similarly, at 48 months of age, children who

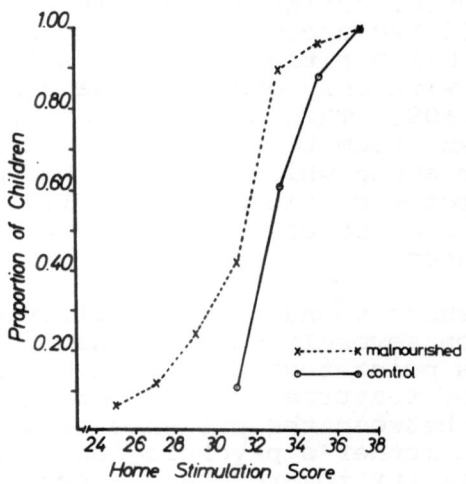

FIGURE 24. Proportion of malnourished and control
children showing different scores of home
stimulation at six months of age.

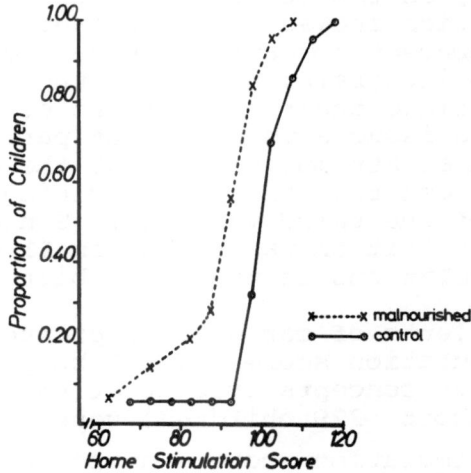

FIGURE 25. Proportion of malnourished and control
children showing different scores in "home
stimulation" at 48 months of age.

had recovered from malnutrition were living in homes
whose scores in home stimulation were quite below those
in which the control children were living. In a range
of scores from 60-120 about 50% of the survivors from
severe clinical malnutrition had home stimulation scores
below 94 points with only one home reaching a score
between 105 and 109. This distribution of scores is
markedly different from that shown by the homes of the
control children among which only one had a score below
95, while four reached values between 110 and 120. These
differences are statistically significant at the 0.01
level of confidence.

The differences found in the quality of home environment between severely malnourished children and
matched controls point toward the convenience of the
analysis of other features of the microenvironment.
The association between the presence of severe clinical
malnutrition and mother's psychological profile, maternal
attitudes, proclivity toward change, concepts on health
and disease, concepts on food and feeding, and family
visiting pattern is under analysis at present in our
laboratory.

Since, on the one hand, the presence of severe
malnutrition was significantly associated with home
stimulation and, on the other hand, survivors of
severe malnutrition showed a significant lag in language bipolar concept formation, it seemed logical to
investigate the interrelations among these three factors
in order to estimate their possible role. As a first
approach to this issue a technique of partial correlation
was employed in an attempt to look at the degree of
association between two variables "holding constant"
the influence of the third variable. Since the number
of cases of malnutrition was rather small we decided to
test for interrelations in the total birth cohort.

The coefficients of correlation product x moment
among home stimulation scores, total body height, and
number of bipolar concepts present at 46 months of age
in the total cohort (229 children) were:

1. home stimulation score - number of bipolar
   concepts = 0.20

2. home stimulation score - total body height
   = 0.23

3. total body height - number of bipolar concepts = 0.26

When the relation between home stimulation and number of bipolar concepts was partialed out for body height the coefficient of correlation dropped from 0.20 to 0.15. When the relation between body height and number of bipolar concepts was partialed out for home stimulation the coefficient changed from 0.26 to 0.23; finally, when number of bipolar concepts was "held constant" the coefficient of correlation between home stimulation and body height changed from 0.23 to 0.19. These results suggest that the association between home stimulation and number of bipolar concepts is mediated, to a good extent, through body height, which in turn holds a significant degree of association with the number of bipolar concepts, independent, to a large extent, of home stimulation. Within the limits of the probabilities given by the magnitude of the coefficients, home stimulation contributes relatively more to body height than to number of bipolar concepts while body height contributes more than home stimulation to the variance of bipolar concepts. Other forms of statistical approach to the problem of the relative contribution of several variables to both the presence of malnutrition and the presence of somatic and mental lags in survivors, such as regression analyses and multivariate analysis of variance, should be tried in order to obtain a more quantitative answer to this subject.

At present, with the results available one can state fairly that: (1) infants prior to the development of severe clinical malnutrition cannot be identified, since they do not differ from the rest of their birth cohort either somatically or behaviorally; (2) the appearance of severe malnutrition seems to be associated, in preindustrial communities, with features of the microenvironment; (3) children who have recovered from severe clinical malnutrition lag behind controls in language development—the poor microenvironmental conditions are not sufficient to fully explain the behavioral lag; (4) the duration of survivors' performance below the values of the matched controls is a point that still lacks an adequate answer.

IMPLICATIONS OF THE FINDINGS

The strong associations found between microenvironmental conditions of the child and the presence of clinical severe malnutrition point, for the first time, toward an explanation of the apparently random occurrence of

severe malnutrition among both families at high risk of
suffering the disease, and children within one of these
families. Why only a few families (1-7%) of all those
with similar low socioeconomic and cultural backgrounds
have children with clinical severe malnutrition, and
only one or two of all the children in the affected
families come all the way down to clinical severe malnutrition, while the other children only show mild-
moderate malnutrition, has been an intriguing question
whose answer has profound public health implications.
The data from our studies seem to indicate that it is a
failure in the microenvironment, the leading factor in
the production of the extremely severe cases of malnutrition. Accordingly, prevention of its occurrence
might be feasible through manipulation of the corresponding variables even without modification of the
macroenvironmental conditions. An intervention model
to test this proposal is being developed in our institu-
tion. If one could prevent third degree malnutrition,
millions of children in the preindustrial societies
could escape the most severe effects of the disease and
its consequences, and the concomitant modification in
parental behavior could start a change in the family
and the society through a better understanding of the
child's needs.

ACKNOWLEDGMENTS

     This work was supported by grants from the Nutrition
Foundation, Inc., the Foundation for Child Development
(formerly Association for the Aid of Crippled Children),
the Van Ameringen Foundation, the Monell Foundation, and
the Hospital del Niño Iman.

REFERENCES

Autret, M., and Behar, M., 1954, "Sindrome pluricarencial
    infantil (Kwashiorkor) and its prevention in Central
    America," FAO Nutritional Series No. 13. Rome, Italy.
Bothe-Antoun, E., Babayan, S., and Harfouche, J. K., 1968,
    "Intellectual development relating to nutritional
    status," J. Trop. Pediatr. 14:112.
Caldwell, B. M., 1967, "Descriptive evaluation of child
    development and of developmental settings," Pediatrics
    40:46.
Champakam, S., Srikantia, S. G., and Gopalan, C., 1968,
    "Kwashiorkor and mental development," Am. J. Clin.
    Nutr. 21:844.

Chase, H. P., and Martin, H. P., 1970, "Undernutrition and child development," New Eng. J. Med. 282:933.

Cravioto, J., 1970, "The complexity of factors involved in protein-calorie malnutrition," Bibl. Nutr. Dieta., No. 14, p. 7, Karger, Basel.

Cravioto, J., and DeLicardie, E. R., 1970, "Mental performance in school-age children: Findings after recovery from early severe malnutrition," Amer. J. Dis. Child. 120:404.

Cravioto, J., and DeLicardie, E. R., 1971a, "The Long-term consequences of protein-calorie malnutrition," Nutr. Rev. 29:107.

Cravioto, J., and DeLicardie, E. R., 1971b, "Infant malnutrition and later learning," in: Progress in Human Nutrition, Vol. 1, S. Margen and N. L. Wilson, eds.) p. 80, Avi Publishing Co., Inc., Westport, Connecticut.

Cravioto, J., and Robles, B., 1962, "The influence of protein-calorie malnutrition on psychological test behavior," Swedish Nutrition Foundation First Symposium on Mild-Moderate Forms of Protein-Calorie Malnutrition," Bastad and Goteborg, August 1962, p. 115.

Cravioto, J., DeLicardie, E. R., and Birch, H. G., 1966, "Nutrition, growth and neurointegrative development: An experimental and ecologic study," Pediatrics 38:319.

Cravioto, J., Birch, H. G., DeLicardie, E. R., and Rosales, L., 1967, "The ecology of infant weight gain in a preindustrial society," Acta Paediatr. Scand. 56:71.

Cravioto, J., Birch, H. G., DeLicardie, E. R., Rosales, L., and Vega, L., 1969, "The ecology of growth and de-velopment in a Mexican preindustrial community. Report 1: Method and findings from birth to one month of age," Monogr. Soc. Res. Child. Dev. 34(5):1 (Serial 129).

Gesell, A., and Amatruda, C., 1947, Developmental Diagnosis: Normal and Abnormal Child Development, Hoeber, New York.

Liang, P. H., Hie, T. T., Jan, O. H., and Giok, L. T., 1967, "Evaluation of mental development in relation to early malnutrition," Am. J. Clin. Nutr. 20:1290.

Monckeberg, F., 1968, "Effect of early marasmic malnu-trition on subsequent physical and psychological devel-opment," in: Malnutrition, Learning, and Behavior, N.S. Scrimshaw and J. E. Gordon, eds.) M.I.T. Press, p. 269.

Pollitt, E., and Granoff, D., 1967, "Mental and motor development of peruvian children treated for severe malnutrition," Rev. Interamericana de Psicologia 1:93.

Yatkin, U. S., and McLaren, D. S., 1970, "The behavioral development of infants recovering from severe malnutri-tion," J. Ment. Defic. Res. 14:25.

NUTRITION, ENVIRONMENT, AND CHILD BEHAVIOR

Merrill S. Read

Growth and Development Branch
National Institute of Child Health
and Human Development
Bethesda, Maryland

Current research is increasingly pointing toward interactions between malnutrition, psychosocial environment, and child development. The papers of Dr. Cravioto and Dr. Pollitt, both of which illustrate ecological or observational types of studies in natural settings, clearly show a clustering of environmental factors which accompany malnutrition (whether seen in rural Mexico or urban United States) which may, in their own right, adversely affect behavioral development. Another large project underway in Guatemala is utilizing a medical-nutritional intervention research design (Canosa et al., 1972). The Guatemalan investigators find two main clusters of environmental factors which influence child development. The first is labeled HOUSE and includes the quality of the house itself, hygienic conditions, crowding, and the human life style that occurs in the house. The second cluster is described as TEACH and is derived from the varied interactions between family members and the individual child, thus contributing to learning experiences. The similarity between these observations and those reported by Cravioto and Pollitt are obvious (Klein et al., 1972).

Not only is the environment of the malnourished child different from that of the well nourished child but also the response of the child himself to his environment is different from normal. Dr. Levitsky (page 75) noted earlier that malnourished rat pups have a

different type of cry and exhibit a low level of demand,
eliciting less response from the mother. Chavez et al.
(1972) have found a very interesting and significant
difference in physical activity between rural Mexican
children born to and nursed by supplemented mothers compared to children born to women not so supplemented. By
the age of two years the supplemented child showed six-
fold more activity than the unsupplemented child; the
child also demanded and received more attention from its
mother. Read (1973a,b) has summarized other data indicating that the heart rate and the arousal level of previously hospitalized malnourished infants are reduced even
after nutritional rehabilitation. Thus the malnourished
child, even following supplementation, differs metaboli-
cally and in the demands he makes of his environment.
This in turn decreases the variety of nature of stimuli
received and ultimately reduces the rate of behavioral
development.

Most of the situations described above are concerned
with moderately severe protein-calorie malnutrition.
This is not seen frequently in the United States, although cases have been documented (Chase et al., 1970),
usually in situations involving family disorganization
or extreme poverty. The more common form of malnutrition
in the U.S. results from a general reduction in calorie
and protein intake leading to moderate growth retardation
rather than to severe stunting (Ten State Survey, 1972).
Such malnutrition is most frequently correlated with
income inadequate to buy sufficient food. Whether this
level of undernutrition influences mental development is
not known; certainly the social and environmental factors
which accompany poverty and malnutrition would be expected to play an increased role in impeding child development under these conditions (Read, 1973b).

The most frequent nutritional problem in the United
States is iron deficiency anemia. This nutritional problem is seen most often in preschool children and in
adolescence and is relatively independent of social
class. The data bearing on anemia and behavior or school
performance have been summarized elsewhere (Read, 1974).
Any effect of anemia on IQ appears to be marginal. However, anemic adolescents do less well on school tasks,
probably due to disruptive behavior in the classroom
rather than to reduced cognitive ability. Similarly,
anemic preschool children exhibit apathetic and irritable
behaviors as well as decreased attentiveness and height-

ened distractability in Head Start settings. Such
behaviors could seriously interfere with learning by
children who are anemic over an extended period of time.

There is still another aspect of food and behavior
which has not been touched upon during this symposium.
I am referring to the impact of hunger on learning and
child development. All too often hunger and malnutrition
are equated in the popular press. They are not the same
at all. Malnutrition results in specific symptoms such
as kwashiorkor, anemia, rickets or indemonstrable growth
retardation. Hunger is a more generalized psychological
and physiological condition arising from a lack of energy
to meet immediate needs. Hunger can be quickly corrected
by feeding; malnutrition requires time for rehabilitation.

It has been estimated that up to a quarter of
America's children may arrive at school without having
had breakfast and may therefore be described as hungry.
There have been practically no well-controlled studies
of hunger or school feeding programs and school performance. Teachers report that hungry children are
apathetic, inattentive, or disruptive in school. The
British Milk Study (1939) noted that a milk-biscuit mid-
morning snack improved school performance during the
school year; biscuits or no-snack groups served as controls. The well known Iowa Breakfast Studies (1962) indicated that providing a standard breakfast in a school
setting beneficially influenced work rate in scholastic
performance in 12- to 14-year-old boys. Several recent
studies in preschool programs have suggested that any
effects of feeding programs which were observed were
more due to benevolent intervention rather than to a
change in nutritional status. These data and related
studies have been summarized elsewhere (Read, 1973b).
In spite of the anecdotal or incomplete nature of the
findings, collectively they suggest that the hungry
child is apathetic, disinterested, and performs less
well in learning situations. Thus hunger forms one
end of the spectrum of effects of malnutrition on child
development. In this case the effect is probably not
due to permanent changes in neurophysiology, but rather,
to the adverse effects on learning from poor interactions between the child and his environment.

Studies are now underway concerning the possible
added benefit of coupling specific educational efforts
with nutritional supplementation to overcome the cumulative effects of prolonged early malnutrition. In

at least one study the results have been most promising
(McKay and Sinisterra, 1973). **In three- to five-year-old**
children living in the slums of Cali, Columbia, a
nutrition-plus-stimulation program has had a better
effect than either a nutrition or a stimulation program
alone. This possibility requires careful study to aid
in designing rehabilitative programs to best meet the
needs of children in the United States as well as in
underdeveloped areas of the world.

        We might summarize all of this research as indica-
ting that the impact of malnutrition is variable depending upon the degree of malnutrition and the nature of the
environment in which the malnutrition occurs. First of
all, severe malnutrition may change the structure and
the function of the **central nervous system; this may**
well be irreversible. As the degree of malnutrition
declines, the importance of the environmental factors
increases, as does the significance of how the child
himself responds to or generates stimuli from the environment around him. In the case of hunger, the response of the child to the world around him may be the
key issue rather than any biological underpinnings at
the neurological level. We must interpret our data
within this continuum in order to generate rational and
promising hypotheses and to formulate effective rehabilitative or preventive programs. And let us also
not forget that long-term successive generations of
chronic undernutrition, as **Dr. Stewart reported to us**
earlier, may have some very serious implications in
terms of the kinds of problems encountered, even in the
United States.

                          REFERENCES

Canosa, C. A., Salomon, J. B., and Klein, R. E., 1972,
  "Field studies of malnutrition and child development-
  the intervention approach: The Guatemala Study," in:
  Nutrition, Growth, and Development of North American
  Indian Children (W. M. **Moore,** M. M. **Silverberg,** and
  M.S. **Read,** eds.), **Publication No.** DHEW (NIH) 72-26,
  U.S. Government Printing Office, Washington, D.C.
The Cereal Institute, Inc., 1962, "A complete summary
  of the Iowa breakfast studies," Chicago.
Chase, H. P., and Martin, H. P., 1970, "Undernutrition
  and child development," New England J. Med. 282 (17):
  933-39.

Chavez, A., Martinez, C., and Bourges, H., 1972, "Nutrition and development of infants from poor rural areas. 2. Nutritional level and physical activity," Nutrition Reports International, 5:139-144.

Klein, R. E., Lester, B. M., Yarbrough, C., and Habicht, J. P., 1972) "Cross-cultural evaluation of human intelligence," in: Lipids, Malnutrition, and the Developing Brain, Ciba Foundation Symposium, Elsevier-Excerpta Medica, Amsterdam.

McKay, H. E., McKay, A., and Sinisterra, C., 1973, "Behavioral intervention studies with malnourished children: A review of experience," in: Nutrition, Development, and Social Behavior (D. J. Kallen, ed.), DHEW Publication (NIH) 73-242, U.S. Government Printing Office, Washington, D.C.

The National Institute for Research in Dairying, 1939, "Milk and nutrition, Part IV: The effects of dietary supplements of pasteurized and raw milk on the growth and health of school children (final report)," Reading, England.

Read, M. S., 1973a, "Malnutrition, hunger and behavior. I. Malnutrition and learning," J. Amer. Diet. Assoc. 63:379-385.

Read, M. S., 1973b, "Malnutrition, hunger and behavior. II. Hunger, school feeding programs and behavior," J. Amer. Diet. Assoc. 63:386-391.

Read, M. S., 1974, "Anemia and behavior," Mod. Probl. Pediat. 14:189-202.

U.S. Dept. H.E.W. Center for Disease Control, 1972, "Highlights, Ten State Nutrition Survey: 1968-1970," Atlanta, Georgia.

THE BIOCHEMICAL ASPECTS
OF NUTRITION AS RELATED
TO MENTAL ILLNESS

INTRODUCTION

Loren R. Mosher

Chief, Center for Studies of Schizophrenia
National Institute of Mental Health
Rockville, Maryland

I am pleased to be here because I think this
meeting is one evidence of the increased level of
interest in the relationship of nutrition to mental
health and to other aspects of health. I think it has
been long overdue. I should perhaps say why I am here.
I am neither a nutritionist nor a basic biochemist; I
have not studied directly the role of vitamins in mental
health. I am here because the Center for Studies of
Schizophrenia has been involved for several years in
the controversy about the usefulness of various vitamins
in the treatment of schizophrenia. This is part of our
role in coordinating the program of NIMH on schizophrenia. The Center disseminates information and con-
ducts program evaluation and development. In a sense,
we attempt to keep abreast of what is going on, what is
reliable information and what is in need of further work.
Based on our evaluations, we stimulate research in certain areas.

For example, we wish to bring the data from NICHD-
supported studies to bear on some of our problems. We
believe it is important to present the available evidence
about the role of vitamins and other nutrients in mental
health and illness to the public and to the scientific
community. Finally, we wish to stimulate and support
research to answer the unanswered questions.

In preparation for this meeting, I made a list of
the possible contributions of the increased interest in
nutrition and mental health for schizophrenia and for

mental illness in general. After that, I listed some
of the possible harmful consequences of this interest.
I believe both should be taken into account in evalua-
ting the situation.

I see two major areas of possible contribution.
The first could be an immediate, rather practical contribution, that is, are vitamins or other nutrients
useful in the treatment of mental disorders in general
and schizophrenia in particular? This is a question
for which we can get at least partial answers relatively
quickly. In the longer run, we would like to know more
about the role of nutrition in psychological growth and
development and its relationship to the development of
mental disorder. In terms of schizophrenia, I think
the most optimistic kind of prediction we can make is
that one or more subgroups of what we now call schizophrenia may be shown to have a nutritional component,
probably interacting with a variety of other things.
Yet, even if only one or two percent of what is now
called schizophrenia is identified as having some kind
of nutritional factor, I think it is well worth the
pursuit.

Now, a bit about the possible adverse consequences.
There is developing a kind of missionary zeal about the
role of nutrition, and vitamins in particular, in mental
illness. What are the possible consequences of this
social movement? First, vitamins, and other substances
as well, can be used indiscriminantly. In the doses
advocated, vitamins no longer act as vitamins, but
rather they act quite like any drug: they have side
effects and dose-related toxicities. In addition to
the potential for direct physical harm are the adverse
consequences associated with the reinforcement of drug-
taking behavior which occurs when persons in authority
advise the use of any drug.

Unfortunately, laymen do not usually obtain complete
scientific information in terms they can understand about
substances they are being encouraged to take. Thus,
calling them natural nutrients and vitamins is both mis-
leading and potentially dangerous. Laymen should know
they are taking a drug, not just a "natural substance."
This distortion plays on ignorance and a natural bias in
favor of innocuous "natural substances" over "drugs"
which might be harmful.

A second major consequence of this missionary zeal is the difficulty it engenders for an objective scientific assessment of the evidence. The zeal of the advocates has resulted in a political process which has impinged on the scientific evaluation process. Thus, doing what we believe is scientifically sound can be interfered with by political pressures. This can, of course, delay obtaining the data we feel is necessary to answer the most pressing questions.

The final problem area associated with this social movement is specific to persons afflicted with schizophrenia. I believe the claims for the usefulness of vitamins in the treatment of schizophrenia are exaggerated. This is bound to lead to great expectations for a vitamin regime. When the schizophrenic does not live up to expectation (i.e., "cure"), he is once again viewed as incurable. Patient, doctor, and family all become disillusioned and disenchanted and withdraw. This is most unfortunate because this state of mutual withdrawal has been shown to perpetuate chronicity in the patient. I think we must be careful when we respond to peoples' need for a simple authoritative answer to a very complicated and difficult life situation, so we do not engender false hopes. It seems to me that this process is occurring with regard to treating schizophrenia with vitamins.

NUTRITION AND PSYCHIATRIC ILLNESS

Seymour S. Kety

**Department of Psychiatry
Harvard Medical School
    and
Director, Psychiatric Research Laboratories
Massachusetts General Hospital
Boston, Massachusetts**

In the early years of this century, as many as 10% of the patients in mental hospitals were there because of the mental disturbances associated with pellagra, a vitamin-deficiency syndrome. The recognition of this as a vitamin deficiency by Goldberger of the Public Health Service and its correction by dietary means produced rapid disappearance of its mental and physical symptoms. Eventually, it was shown that the important agent that was deficient was nicotinic acid. Here was an instance of an important mental illness where research eventually demonstrated a biochemical disturbance as its cause, leading to successful therapy. This remarkable discovery also set the stage for considerable speculation and less well supported claims for the operation of vitamin deficiencies in a variety of other mental illnesses whose etiologies were still obscure. Of such illnesses, the most important is undoubtedly schizophrenia.

Research in schizophrenia has been plagued for many decades by a number of problems and sources of error, methodological and intellectual pitfalls. Like cancer, schizophrenia is tragic and frightening. It affects large numbers of the population and their families and for this reason undoubtedly has motivated many serious scientists to devote themselves to its study. Also like cancer, it has spawned a number of extravagant, premature and pseudoscientific therapeutic claims. The typical

schizophrenic patient who has been used in biochemical
studies for a number of decades is often a chronically
ill patient who has been institutionalized in mental
hospitals for five, ten, even twenty years. Chronic
hospitalization in overcrowded, inadequately funded
institutions produces certain changes in the patient
which are not characteristic of the illness and are
irrelevant to it. These changes are psychological,
physical, and nutritional. A major task for the scientist is to separate the changes which are secondary to
institutionalization from the primary and characteristic
phenomena. The history of biochemical research in
psychiatry is replete with instances in which important
etiological claims were made for a biochemical finding
in institutionalized schizophrenics which was not appropriately separated from the simple, chronic effects of
hospitalization or the dietary inadequacies associated
with it. For example, in the earlier literature of this
century, a number of researchers reported changes in
carbohydrate metabolism and in hepatic function of
schizophrenic patients. Horwitt, recognizing that many
of the vitamins were important cofactors in carbohydrate
metabolism, undertook an examination of simple vitamin
deficiencies which occurred in mental hospital patients
and indicated that many of the biochemical changes which
had been attributed to schizophrenia were simply the result of mild vitamin deficiencies. He also showed that
a dietary intake which was deficient in protein could
produce some of the other biochemical changes and indications of mild hepatic dysfunction which had been found
in many schizophrenics. Such changes could be made to
disappear by dietary restitution without affecting the
mental status.

In 1956, in the Laboratory of Clinical Science at
the National Institute of Mental Health, my associates
and I undertook a long-term study of the biochemical and
biological aspects of schizophrenia. We attempted to
remove or control as many of these nondisease variables
as possible. Patients who were free of demonstrable
medical illness were selected from the state hospitals
of Maryland and the District of Columbia. They were
housed in a ward at the Clinical Center, where appropriate psychotherapeutic milieu therapy could be in-
stituted and where an adequate dietary intake was maintained. The remarkable thing about the studies which
were conducted with these patients and a suitable group
of normal volunteers was the difficulty in differentiating
the schizophrenic patients biochemically from the normal

volunteers. Among the most interesting studies in that
laboratory was the work of McDonald and his associates
on vitamin C and schizophrenia. This was prompted by a
report by a young Swedish biochemist that DPP, a dye
which is colorless in its reduced form and becomes red
on oxidation, turned pink when added to the serum of
schizophrenics. About this time, a group in New Orleans
reported that when epinephrine was added to the serum
of schizophrenics, it was oxidized much more rapidly
than in normal plasma. Hence it was surmised that the
important agent involved in this kind of oxidation in
the serum is ceruloplasmin. Holmberg and Lorell had
described ceruloplasmin some years before these studies,
and had shown that it is a mild oxidase present in normal plasma and that it is capable of oxidizing DPP and
epinephrine, among numerous other substrates. What
Holmberg and Lorell also pointed out, however, was that
another substance in the plasma, ascorbic acid or vitamin C, acts to inhibit this enzymatic activity. McDonald,
feeling that many schizophrenics might be suffering from
a deficiency of ascorbic acid on a dietary basis, surmised that low plasma ascorbic acid might explain the
apparent increase in ceruloplasmin activity found in
schizophrenic patients. He examined the serum of
schizophrenic patients who had been maintained on a good
diet for its ability to oxidize adrenalin or DPP. The
reaction he obtained was normal. He studied some of the
staff who were not drinking a glass of orange juice each
morning and found that some of them gave an abnormal
reaction. He went to state hospitals and examined patients who had been institutionalized for long periods
of time and found that most were positive reactors. When
he analyzed the blood of the patients and subjects for
ascorbic acid, he found an excellent correlation between
reduced levels of ascorbic acid in a blood sample and its
ability to oxidize epinephrine or DPP. McDonald pursued
this further and added ascorbic acid to the diet of the
patients in the state hospitals, raised their ascorbic
acid levels and obtained normal serum oxidase tests. He
also put normal volunteers on a low-ascorbic-acid diet,
and showed that these normal subjects now gave a positive
test supposedly indicative of schizophrenia. When he
restored the dietary ascorbic acid, the tests again
showed normal reactions. In none of this was there any
change in the mental status of the normals or of the
schizophrenics. From these data, it is quite clear that
these findings can be attributed to a simple dietary
deficiency--secondary to institutionalization--which in
fact had nothing to do with schizophrenia, and which can

readily be corrected by supplementing the diet with
vitamin C. This made the blood test negative, but
unfortunately did not affect the schizophrenia.

Another example of a presumed biochemical disturbance in schizophrenia which has been thought by some
to be caused by a relative vitamin deficiency has to do
with the claims that large doses of nicotinic acid or
its amide can effectively treat schizophrenia. The
history of this observation is an interesting one.
Cantoni described, on the basis of very competent fundamental biochemistry, a process which came to be known
as biological transmethylation. In this reaction, the
amino acid methionine is converted to an activated
form, S-adenosylmethionine. With the aid of appropriate
enzymes this activated methionine is capable of trans-
ferring its methyl group to certain substrates. It was
quickly realized that many substances important in
physiology, for example, epinephrine, are formed in the
body by a process in which S-adenosylmethionine transfers its methyl group to an appropriate substrate. In
the case of epinephrine, the substrate is norepinephrine.

In 1962, Harley-Mason, in an appendix to a paper
by Osmond and Smythies, put forward the interesting
hypothesis that biological transmethylation might be
disturbed in schizophrenia, permitting the accumulation
of toxic substances that could possibly account for the
hallucinations which are common in that disorder.
Harley-Mason was impressed by the fact that many of the
known hallucinogens are methylated compounds and that
at least one of them is a methylated congener of dopamine, i.e., mescaline, which is dopamine with three
methoxy groups around its ring. He suggested the interesting possibility that catecholamines could be O-meth-
ylated in the body by biological transmethylation. He
thus predicted the discovery that Axelrod made five years
later: O-methylation is an important mechanism for de-
grading catecholamines. He also postulated that perhaps
some normal metabolites may be methylated to form hallucinogens and that these may accumulate in the schizophrenic due to an inability to detoxify them, thereby
causing some of the symptoms of schizophrenia.

In 1954, Hoffer, Osmond and Smythies suggested that
an abnormal metabolism of epinephrine could explain the
symptoms of schizophrenia by being converted to adrenochrome, an oxidation product of epinephrine which was
well known to occur _in_ _vitro_ and which accounts for the

pink color which epinephrine shows after exposure to the air in aqueous solutions. This idea had some rather attractive features. It could account for the convergence of genetic and experiential factors in schizophrenia. It was compatible with the idea that there was some genetic defect in the metabolism of epinephrine but that this would not necessarily show itself until there was a huge outpouring of epinephrine as a result of life stress. This could overwhelm the incompetent enzymatic machinery normally able to degrade epinephrine and cause an influx of adrenochrome into the blood stream, producing the symptoms of schizophrenia. Hoffer and Osmond extracted some adrenochrome and injected it into each other and satisfied themselves that it was capable of producing hallucinations.

Attempts to validate the adrenochrome hypothesis were, however, unsuccessful. A number of other groups in controlled studies injected adrenochrome into volunteers and did not observe hallucinogenic properties. I find it rather interesting to read Hoffer's description of the history of the adrenochrome hypothesis. In a paper in <u>Point</u> <u>Counterpoint</u> entitled, "The Orthomolecular Treatment for Schizophrenia," published in December, 1972, he writes: "In 1952, Osmond and I established the adrenochrome hypothesis of schizophrenia." This seems to be something of a hyperbole since the hypothesis has not yet been established. He goes on to state: "The only serious research to examine the idea outside of our own work came from Altschule's laboratory." Altschule had put forth an "aminochrome" hypothesis (aminochrome being a somewhat larger group of chromatogenic amine compounds of which adrenochrome is one), but that hypothesis has not yet been confirmed or widely accepted. I find it even more difficult to understand how Hoffer could write in 1972 that this was the only serious research, outside of his own, which examines this idea, because it is quite contradictory to what actually occurred. I would like to describe some serious research which attempted to test the adrenochrome hypothesis. It was published more than ten years ago and Hoffer appears to have forgotten about it.

In the Laboratory of Clinical Science, some of us were attracted by the adrenochrome hypothesis and proceeded to think about how it might be tested. Earlier, McDonald had shown that the increased oxidation of adrenalin by the serum of some schizophrenics could be accounted for merely in terms of ascorbic acid deficiency

which nonschizophrenics could show equally well. We were
also aware of the lack of ability of other workers to
confirm the hallucinogenic properties of adrenochrome.
But the really crucial test of the hypothesis would be
to examine the metabolism of epinephrine in schizophrenic
individuals. Now that was rather difficult to do in the
mid-50's because little was known about the normal metabolism of epinephrine, let alone its metabolism in schizophrenia. One way of approaching this would be to ad-
minister labelled epinephrine with sufficient amounts of
the label to permit isolation and identification of its
metabolites in the urine. We had some tritiated epinephrine synthesized because that would give us the specific
activity required. But more important, Axelrod, who was
a member of the laboratory, became interested in the
metabolism of epinephrine. Stimulated by a paper by
Armstrong and his associates reporting an interesting
new metabolite in the urine of a patient with pheno-
chromocytoma, Axelrod postulated that in the metabolism
of epinephrine, two processes would be involved--deamin-
ation and O-methylation. He then characterized the enzyme
for O-methylation and predicted the existence of a sub-
stanial number of metabolites on a theoretical basis.
Those metabolites were then identified in the urine of
animals.

On the basis of Axelrod's careful delineation of the
normal metabolism of epinephrine and the methods which
he had developed for the isolation and characterization
of these various compounds, it was possible for LaBrosse
and others in the laboratory to use the tritiated epinephrine to carry out a study on the metabolism of epinephrine in a group of 12 schizophrenic and 12 normal
individuals. There was no gross difference in the metabolism of epinephrine between the normals and the schizophrenics and no adrenochrome was found in the urine of
either group. That was certainly serious research and I
cannot explain why Dr. Hoffer failed to cite it.

However, on the basis of the transmethylation
hypothesis and the adrenochrome hypothesis, Hoffer and
Osmond developed the idea that if transmethylation in
schizophrenics could be impeded, formation of adrenochrome might be prevented. They thought of the rather
ingenious idea of using nicotinic acid or nicotinamide,
which they assumed to be methyl acceptors, to divert
the methylation processes from producing hallucinogens
to producing innocuous n-methyl nicotinamide which would
then be excreted. They tested the ability of nicotinic

acid or nicotinamide to affect schizophrenia and reported very dramatic benefits. It is rather interesting
that these results came about because later work by
Baldessarini and Kopin indicated that nicotinamide or
nicotinic acid were not very effective as methyl acceptors in the brain. A substantial number of carefully
controlled studies by a number of other groups have
failed to support the earlier claims that nicotinic acid
or its amide are effective in the treatment of schizophrenia. Yet that has not dampened the enthusiasm of
the proponents of that treatment whose claims have become more and more extravagant. For example, "It
follows," writes Dr. Hoffer, "that enrichment of our
food with vitamin B[3] which is nicotinic acid will prevent most cases of pellagra or of schizophrenia from
becoming manifest. I estimate that one gram per day
started early in life will protect most of us." In
another instance: "There is no doubt that a major proportion of schizophrenics recover on vitamin B[3]." Reporting a controlled evaluation of this treatment, Dr.
Hoffer wrote: "Patients on nicotinic acid in all the
groups were better off. These results are so strikingly
different that no statistical tests are required." In
more recent years, he and his associates have disre-
garded controlled studies and justify the treatment on
the basis of testimonial reports by some of the physicians or patients who have used it. Their treatment has
also changed over the past decade to include a large
number of vitamins in large dosages and when the phenothiazine drugs became established as effective therapy
in schizophrenia throughout the world, those too were
incorporated in the treatment regimen.

In 1968, support came to this school of treatment
from an unexpected quarter. Linus Pauling published a
paper in Science which coined the term "orthomolecular
psychiatry" and presented an interesting hypothesis.
He suggested that the notion of a "minimal daily requirement" for vitamins was invalid because of the
genetic variability of the population. Thus what may
be an optimal intake for one individual may be grossly
inadequate for another. One cannot argue with that concept. In fact, Rosenberg and others have described a
number of well defined monogenic neurological disorders
with demonstrable and specific defects in the utilization
of particular vitamins which respond dramatically and
promptly when that vitamin is administered in large
doses. The clinical symptoms reappear quite promptly
when the vitamin is withdrawn. It is certainly possible,

as Pauling goes on to suggest, that some mental illnesses
and some forms of schizophrenia may eventually be shown
to be the result of a similar disturbance. What is
lacking thus far, however, is acceptable evidence in
support of that hypothesis.

Dr. Morris A. Lipton has headed a task force of
the American Psychiatric Association which is examining
the basis of the megavitamin therapy and reviewing the
claims of its proponents versus more than a dozen controlled studies which do not support these claims.
Their report finds little to substantiate either the
theoretical basis or the empirical value of megavitamin
therapy and questions the credibility of some of its
proponents.

There is every reason to continue fundamental research on the relationship of particular vitamins to
the metabolism of the brain and to mental state and to
look for disturbances in the utilization of specific
vitamins in particular psychiatric conditions. These
relationships have not yet been demonstrated, however,
and it seems unwise, on the basis of the evidence available, to advocate widespread or indiscriminate use of
an assortment of vitamins in large and possibly harmful
dosages with patients suffering from one or another form
of schizophrenia.

PREMORBID ADJUSTMENT AND RESPONSE TO NICOTINIC ACID

John R. Wittenborn

Director, Interdisciplinary Research Center
Rutgers University
New Brunswick, New Jersey

INTRODUCTION

Some years ago the Rutgers Interdisciplinary Research Center received what then seemed to be a very
large grant to study the hypothesis that nicotinic
acid in large doses was effective in the treatment of
schizophrenia (Hoffer et al., 1957). The research
plan for this comprehensive study provided for a sample
of 100 patients on treatment for the course of two years.
All of the patients were new admissions at the New Jersey
State Hospital at Marlboro. All were males and very few
of them could be described as chronic patients. The
median duration of prior hospitalization during the
preceding five years was 7 1/2 weeks.

The patients were assigned on a random double-blind
basis to either a nicotinic acid-high dosage regimen of
3000 mg per day, or to a control regimen of 6 mg per day.
60% of the patients were assigned to the experimental
group and 40% to the control group. Such a ratio permitted the anticipated scrutiny of the differences among
those patients receiving the high dosage regimen.

It is very difficult to keep schizophrenic patients
on treatment for two years, particularly in this era
when after a few months, if not weeks, almost all patients become outpatients. Accordingly, provisions were
made to follow the patients closely in the community
subsequent to their discharge from the hospital.

Psychiatrists and psychologists saw them at least once a month for examinations, and social workers called at their homes and talked with family informants to assess and record their adjustment within the community.

Of special importance was the task of keeping the outpatients on medication and assessing their status from the standpoint of any metabolic disturbances that might occur. Disturbed carbohydrate metabolism and enteritis had been anticipated when the study was planned. Neither of these problems occurred. A kind of pigmentation which appeared at first to resemble an acanthosis nigricans did occur in about one third of the patients treated with high dosage nicotinic acid. In every case this dermatosis was only a superficial involvement which never appeared before the fourth month and disappeared after treatment had been reduced or terminated for a few weeks. The literature contains several articles documenting this reaction to continued high dosage nicotinic acid (Brown and Winkelmann, 1968). None of these was found in the psychiatric literature, despite the fact that there is substantial literature describing the use of nicotinic acid in the treatment of psychiatric patients.

METHODS AND RESULTS

General Response

The research plan provided for a large number of assessments at regular intervals. Assessments involved various rating scales to measure symptomatic aberrations, and inventories and other such devices to indicate subjective state were used. Repeated intensive assays of outpatient adjustment were made by the social workers on the basis of interviews with family informants. Psychomotor tests were used by psychologists.

No differences between the two treatment groups were found over time, i.e., there were virtually no significant differences and any distinguishing trend seemed to suggest that the patients in the experimental group (high dosage nicotinic acid) were slightly, but not significantly, worse than the patients in the control group (Wittenborn et al., 1973).

In general, patients who have an average rating
above 0.50 on the various scales which comprise the
depressive retardation cluster of the Wittenborn Psychiatric Rating Scale (WPRS) are considered to have a clinically appreciable degree of depression. 45 of the 47
patients in the experimental group and 27 of the 28 patients in the control group had such a symptom level at
pretreatment. The portion of patients having a significant level of depressive retardation at the successive
assessment periods is presented in Figure 1 as a percent of the patients who had such a level of this symptom
complex at the beginning of treatment. At six months
there is a substantial drop in both the experimental
group and the control group, and this reduction in the
prevalence of depressive retardation is maintained
throughout the course of treatment. No difference between the two groups emerged during the course of treatment.

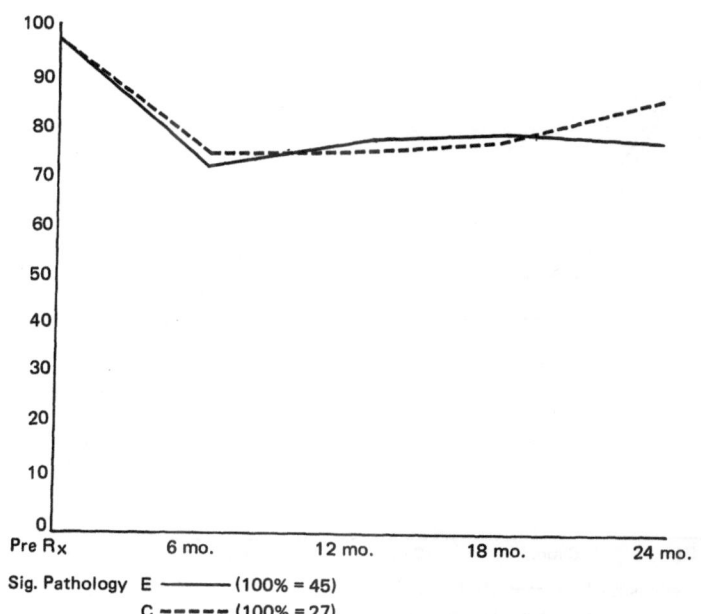

FIGURE 1. Percent of patients with $\overline{X}$ pretreatment rating
of at least 0.50 who had a subsequent $\overline{X}$ rating
above 0.50, WPRS Depressive Retardation.

Figure 2 indicates the portion of patients having
a significant degree of another symptom complex, schizophrenic excitement. At six months there was a substantial
diminution (approximately 50%) for the two treatment
groups. This diminution continued so that at 24 months
about 30% of both groups showed a significant degree of
schizophrenic excitement. This kind of analysis is
based on the portion of the sample showing a qualitatively
significant level of this psychopathology at a given time
and does not quantify the level of severity.

Other relevant symptom complexes were examined and
showed similar trends. For example, for paranoia and
hebephrenia there was a large drop in the portion of patients having an average rating above 0.50 at six months,
and there was further subsequent diminution. There was
no important and persisting separation between the two
treatment groups.

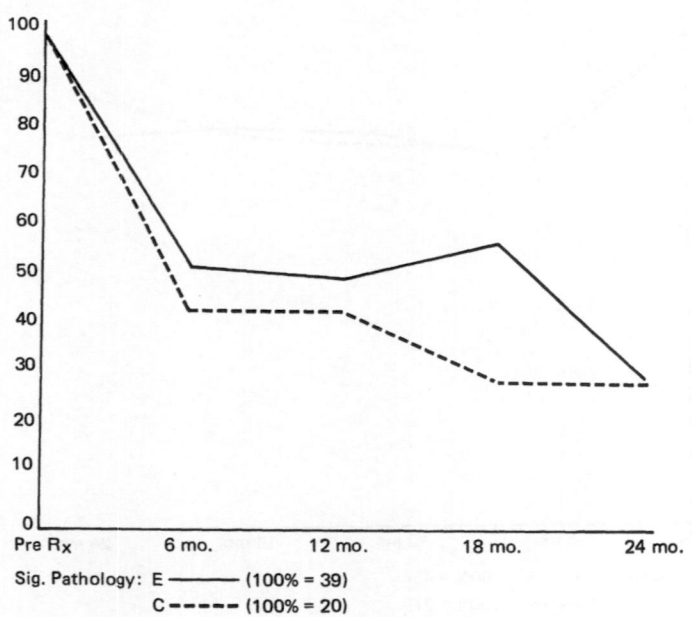

FIGURE 2. Percent of patients with $\overline{X}$ pretreatment rating
          of at least 0.50 who had a subsequent $\overline{X}$ rating
          above 0.50, WPRS Schizophrenic Excitement.

Differential Response

Analyses currently in progress are based upon the
75 patients who remained in treatment for a period of
two years. Data were examined from the standpoint of
seeking some identifiable group of persons for whom
nicotinic acid might be advantageous. The goal of this
search was to find a kind of differential discriminator--
a factor that might be associated with reduced pathology
in the experimental group and with persisting or even
increased pathology in the control group. As an illus-
tration, Table I shows cyclothymic history to be a
differential discriminator with favorable implications
for the nicotinic acid group and unfavorable implications
for the control group.

TABLE I. Premorbid Cyclothymia as a Differential
Discriminator between Experimental and Control
Groups with Respect to Schizophrenic Excitement
at 24 Months

Cyclothymic	Experimental		Control		
	$\bar{X}$	n	$\bar{X}$	n	t
yes	.22	(10)	.69	(6)	2.91
no	.56	(37)	.38	(22)	1.58
Total	.49	(47)	.45	(28)	1.18
t	2.10				

$$F_{Rows \times Col.} = 7.39$$

Items from the social worker's pretreatment inquiry
descriptive of the patient's premorbid adjustment were
correlated with the criteria represented by symptom-rating
scores. These correlations were computed for every time
interval. Upon inspection, it appeared that the items
from the social worker's inquiry that showed a significant
interaction with the experimental group versus control
group distinction seemed to have something in common.
The common element of meaning which gave plausibility

suggested that the items could be combined in a simple
additive manner to form a kind of differential discriminator score, a predictor score. These items are listed
in Table II.

Figure 3 shows the correlations between the differentially discriminating positive predictor score and
schizophrenic excitement, hebephrenia, paranoia, and
depressive retardation, respectively, at pretreatment,
6, 12, 18, and 24 months. The trends are relatively
stable when one considers the fact that these are correlation coefficients for what must be fairly unreliable
measures and for small samples.

TABLE II. Differentially Discriminating Items Comprising
          the Positive Predictor Score

---

1. Patient does not prefer to be by himself.

2. Patient does not withdraw as relationships become
   close.

3. Patient has had positive relationships.

4. Patient has sought dependent relationships.

5. Patient feels that he is attractive to females.

6. Family approves of spouse.

7. Spouse is not ridiculing.

8. Spouse is not rigidly demanding.

9. Patient has supported himself.

10. Patient feels that development of his talents was
    suppressed.

11. Patient has a sense of humor.

12. Patient is cyclothymic.

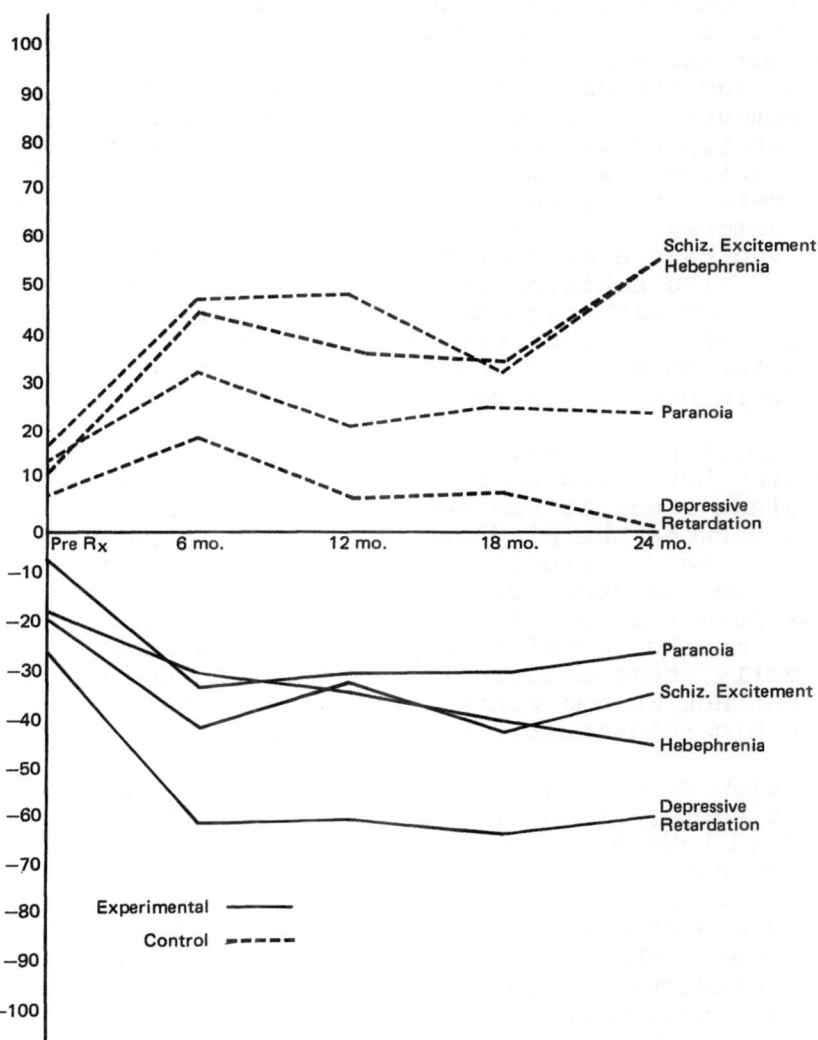

FIGURE 3. Correlation between positive predictor score
and WPRS scores of symptomatic severity.

Since the correlations at pretreatment time are quite low, the substantial subsequent relationships between the predictor score and the various criteria scores are emergent treatment-dependent relationships. During the course of treatment, presumably during the first 6 months, something has accrued to affect the magnitude and the direction of the relationship in the two treatment groups. The data have been scrutinized most carefully to discover any possible artifacts in these relationships, and none has been found. If this kind of relationship can be cross-validated by an independent sample, it would suggest that there may be some persons who have a dissociative type of psychosis which might look like schizophrenia and who could be beneficially treated with high dosages of nicotinic acid. It would suggest also that the illness of these patients might follow an adverse course relative to other patients if they were not so treated.

Although no cross-validating studies of these relationships have been undertaken, within the scope of the original study it was possible to examine the relationship between the predictor score and outpatient adjustment. The relationships between the positive predictor score and good outpatient adjustment as indicated by items from the social worker's follow-up inquiry at 12 and 24 months revealed an interesting pattern. Specifically, this association is found in the experimental group, but not in the control group. The follow-up items showing this relationship tell their own story (Table III).

In view of the relationships found for the positive predictor score, it is of interest to ask the question, "What would have happened if niacin had been given to only those patients who had a high positive predictor score, e.g., above 0.60, and who also had a clinically appreciable degree of the symptom-complex under question?" Figure 4 shows the per cent of patients with both a high positive predictor score and a mean WPRS depressive retardation pretreatment rating of at least 0.50 who had a subsequent mean rating above 0.50. It is apparent that there is some distinction between the two treatment groups starting at 6 months and continuing through 24 months. Figure 5 shows a similar relationship for schizophrenic excitement. In the nicotinic acid group there is a drop to about 30% which starts at 6 months and continues through 18 months. By 24 months only about 10% of the patients in the nicotinic acid group had such ratings.

TABLE III. Correlations between Follow-up Items and a Positive Predictor Score for Experimental Patients (E) and Control Patients (C)

Follow-up Social Work Item	12 Months		24 Months	
	E	C	E	C
Patient does not feel sorry for himself.	35	01	35	-19
Patient does not lack confidence in ordinary tasks.	45	14	51	02
Patient does not procrastinate.	37	-06	46	14
Patient does not object to throwing things away.	72	23	31	-01
Patient seems generally happy.	31	04	30	00
Patient does not prefer to be by himself.	37	21	31	24
Patient does not mind meeting new people.	39	12	39	29
Patient is a particularly understanding person.	28	17	52	17
Patient can keep friends.	50	-03	36	-04
Patient does go out socially.	31	-08	47	-14
Patient has supported himself.	34	04	51	-19
Patient has started new social hobbies, avocations.	34	-27	38	-21
Patient did get a job.	31	-03	47	-14

FIGURE 4.

Percent of patients with depressive retardation showing both a high positive predictor score and a $\bar{X}$ pretreatment rating of at least 0.50 who had a subsequent $\bar{X}$ rating above 0.50.

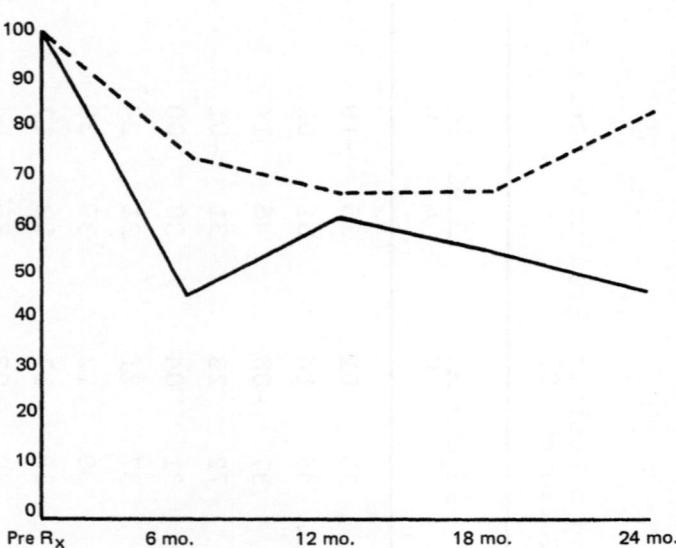

Positive Predictor and Sig. Pathology: E' ——— (100% = 13)
                                         C' ----- (100% = 12)

FIGURE 5.

Percent of patients with schizophrenic excitement showing both a high positive predictor score and a $\bar{X}$ pretreatment rating of at least 0.50 who had a subsequent $\bar{X}$ rating above 0.50.

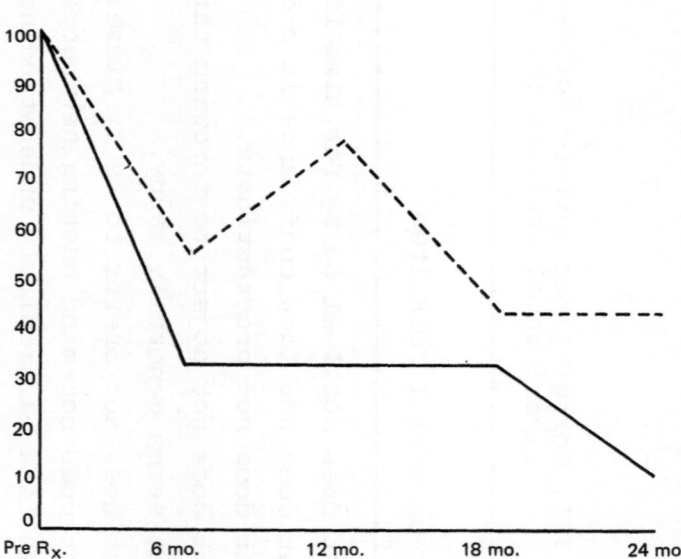

Positive Predictor and Sig. Pathology: E'——— (100% = 9)
                                           C'------ (100% = 9)

In contrast, the control group drops to about 55% at 6 months and to 45% by 24 months. There is a similar but greater contrast for the paranoia and hebephrenia WPRS scores at 24 months, Figures 6 and 7 respectively.

FIGURE 6.

Percent of patients with paranoia showing both a high positive predictor score and a $\bar{X}$ pretreatment rating of at least 0.50 who had a subsequent $\bar{X}$ rating above 0.50.

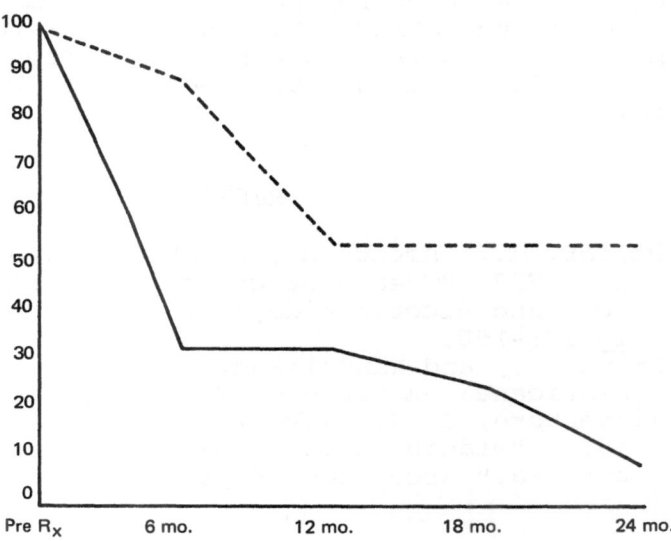

Positive Predictor and Sig. Pathology: E' ——— (100% = 12)
C' ------ (100% = 9)

FIGURE 7.

Percent of patients with hebephrenia showing both a high positive predictor score and a $\bar{X}$ pretreatment rating of at least 0.50 who had a subsequent $\bar{X}$ rating above 0.50.

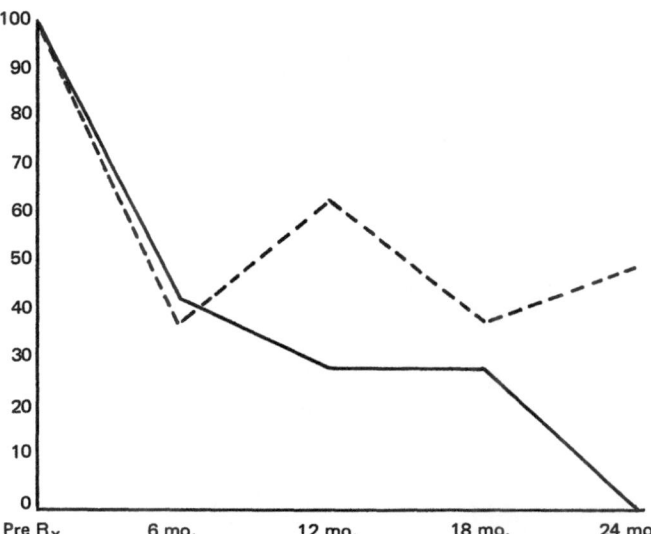

Positive Predictor and Sig. Pathology: E' ——— (100% = 7)
C' ------ (100% = 8)

CONCLUSIONS

On the basis of the present results, it is difficult
to sustain a claim that nicotinic acid is a <u>generally</u>
useful treatment for patients who come to hospitals with
a condition called schizophrenia. Nevertheless, there
may be some persons who have psychoses of a dissociative
nature for whom this treatment could be an important
gain.

REFERENCES

Hoffer, A., Osmond, H., Callbeck, M. J., and Kahan,
    I., 1957, "Treatment of schizophrenia with nicotinic
    acid and nicotinamide," J. Clin. Exp. Psychopathol.
    <u>18</u>:131-158.
Brown, J., and Winkelmann, R. K., 1968, "Acanthosis
    nigricans: A study of 90 cases," Medicine <u>47</u>:33-51.
Wittenborn, J. R., Weber, E. S. P., and Brown, M.,
    1973, "Niacin in the long-term treatment of schizo-
    phrenia," Arch. Gen. Psychiat. <u>28</u>:308-315.

WORKSHOP ON NUTRITION

INTRODUCTION

Mervyn Susser

Chairman, Department of Epidemiology
Columbia University
New York, N.Y.

As moderator for the session, I will pose some problems that might be covered in the discussion. Later I will speak about the Dutch famine studies we have now completed, if it seems appropriate and useful. Studies of the effects of human nutrition on development are extremely difficult, and most answers are tentative.

A first problem is the measurement of input, that is, the establishment of the actual nutritional intake of the subjects and their controls. In human studies we are generally working on assumptions in regard to input.

A second problem is a general experimental problem, a human research problem, that is acute in nutritional studies. The problem is to isolate the nutritional input variable from all those other factors that surround it, and within which it is embedded. The problem was illustrated earlier by Drs. Pollitt and Cravioto as well as by Seymour Kety, in his discussion of the megavitamin problem.

If we are going to deal effectively with these questions in human research, we must sharpen research design. We have to use multivariate analysis, and also we must be discriminating in our categorization of outcomes. In particular, we must discriminate carefully between effects at different levels of organization in the hierarchy of systems, and there Dr. Cravioto has given us a lead. It is important to be clear when we are

talking about the organic level and its impairment, which
requires clinical and pathological measures. There is
no one-to-one relationship between the organic level of
impairment and the higher level of function. Functional
disability requires psychological measures of different
kinds. A third level of organization is social, and
expressed as demonstrable social handicap. Handicap requires measures in terms of social roles and social relationships. Again, there is not a one-to-one relationship between psychological dysfunction and social role.
When we examine each of these levels, we are looking at
separate but interrelated outcomes. In all these re-
spects, we have gained much greater sophistication over
the last several years.

    Some of the problems we face are frank conflicts
between the results of different studies on the same
question. We are still confronted with the issue of
whether nutritional deprivation affects mental performance in later life. This question is open for nutritional
deprivation both prenatally and postnatally. Our own
Dutch famine study gave us a negative result with regard
to the effect of __prenatal__ starvation on the mental
competence and health states of young men. In addition,
some recent studies like Hansen's sibling control study
in Capetown gave a negative result with regard to the
effect of __postnatal__ malnutrition on later mental competence and growth. Hansen detected no differences between
patients admitted with acute nutritional failure who were
followed over several years, and their siblings. On the
other hand, a contradictory result can be found in the
Jamaican study of the late Herbert Birch, Margaret Hertzig,
Stephen Richardson, and Jack Tizard, also with a sibling control. The questions to be resolved, then, are
really quite difficult. One can argue, and I think it
is reasonable to argue, that in Hansen's study the siblings could have been as malnourished as the index cases,
and that what differentiates patients and siblings is
not malnutrition but admission to the hospital. But admission to hospital may be for reasons quite unconnected
with nutrition, like the breakup of family, or social
mobility and marital mobility.

    This explanation of confounding can also be applied
to the Jamaican work of Garrow and Pike, and their
failure to find an effect of early kwashiorkor on height
among cases and their siblings. On the other hand, the
Birch studies in Jamaica do find a difference, and here
one can make the same criticism of a study that produced

the opposite result. Again, that is, what may differentiate the outcomes between cases and their siblings could
be their hospital experience. I think personally that
the gradient of results in the Jamaican studies is convincing, particularly in rural children; urban children
did not give such clear results. The Capetown studies
involve urban children and maybe the difference lies
there. The difference in the results in Jamaica and
Capetown, thus, could be an urban/rural difference, and
the urban/rural difference might point to the social
environment in interaction with the nutritional factor.

Another question I would like to hear discussed is
that of timing of the measurement of the deferred manifestations of malnutrition, and also timing of the
nutritional insult. Differences in the time of measurement may resolve some of the conflicts in results. In
our Dutch study we looked at adults, after a prenatal
nutritional insult, and found no effect. Herbert Birch
and his colleagues timed their measurements of manifes-
tation at about 11 years of age, after a nutritional insult under two years of age, and found some effect. The
manifestational differences in those who had the acute
nutritional insult may have been still greater at age 3
or 4 than at age 11. In other words, we may be dealing
with a diminishing effect. The effect might disappear
as the pressures of socialization introduce more environmental input and overwhelm the early nutritional experience of the affected infants.

The question of the critical period also needs
sharp discussion, because there are many conflicts in
the data. We have the results of McCance and Widdowson,
Winick's work on the critical period in animals, and
his work with Rosso on human autopsies; all these suggest the presence of a critical period. Cravioto's work
with Robles in infants also suggests that early exposure
to malnutrition is necessary to produce an ultimate
effect on mental competence. On the other hand, Birch,
Hertzig, Richardson, and Tizard could find no indication
of a critical period in the Jamaican study. The studies
of Chase and Martin at Denver show almost the opposite;
that is, the children who were admitted after about ten
months of age had more severe effects than those admitted at four months. Duration of malnutrition could
be a plausible explanation of the Denver result. That
is, duration of exposure might have been more important
than time of exposure. Finally, we were unable in our
Dutch study to isolate a prenatal critical period effect

on later mental performance. On the other hand, we did
detect such a critical period in the third trimester,
in relation to fetal growth and mortality, and another,
in the first trimester, in relation to central nervous
system organogenesis and mortality.

These are the questions that I am hoping we shall
discuss.

SOME COMMENTS ON THE EFFECTS OF MALNUTRITION ON

BRAIN FUNCTION

David B. Coursin

Director of Research
St. Joseph's Hospital
Lancaster, Pennsylvania

For the record, I would like to commend Mr. Kittay, his Foundation, and its Board for their recognition of psychiatry as an important dimension of medicine. I understand that the Foundation is specifically focused on psychiatry per se and that their interest in malnutrition is somewhat secondary. However, they are clearly aware of the important long-range potential effects of malnutrition on the psychiatric dimensions of life. Furthermore, I would like to congratulate all of the speakers for their fine contributions to the meetings.

I would like to comment briefly on a number of important aspects of the broad problem of the effects of malnutrition on brain function. Evidence now available indicates that diet and environmental conditions are biologically inseparable in their multiplicative effects on the developing brain and its performance. This has been particularly evident in severe malnutrition (i.e., kwashiorkor and marasmus) that occurs in less than 10% of populations with serious nutritional risk. Furthermore, it appears likely that lesser but somewhat similar consequences may occur in those who have experienced mild to moderate malnutrition.

Recent research indicates that both deficiencies in nutrient intake and deficiencies in environmental stimulation can produce a somewhat similar impairment of behavior and performance. While the mechanisms are not well understood, it appears that they do not involve

permanent major abnormalities in brain structure and
composition but rather derive from alterations in the
individual's activity, alertness, attention, experiential interaction, and emotionality. These factors
individually and collectively may reduce normal capabilities in subnormal performance.

A number of types of studies have been undertaken
in human populations in order to explore the various
aspects of this problem. Various designs have been
used including cross-sectional, longitudinal, and over-
lapping. Each provides particular kinds of information
with the recent focus of research centering on longitudinal perspective studies. These have been multidisciplinary in structure and have endeavored to document
most of the major dietary and environmental factors
that may be involved in this problem.

Two major types of studies have been undertaken--
ecological and intervention. Dr. Cravioto has pursued
the ecological approach most productively and has reported to us on some of his findings. This method
provides an understanding of the nature and course of
malnutrition in a population at risk with a minimum of
outside influence.

A second approach is that of intervention in which
separate but similar populations--one with nutritional
supplementation and one without--are compared. Dr. Klein
in Guatemala has reported on the kinds of information
that can be derived from such studies. In addition,
work by Dr. Chow in Taiwan and by Dr. Chavez in Mexico
has further extended the application of this approach.

It has been evident from this meeting as well as
others that all of the disciplines concerned with the
study of the effects of malnutrition on the brain have
limitations in the specificity and sensitivity of tools
for measurement that can be applied to these problems.
In some disciplines, parameters can be readily quanti-
fied with a reasonable degree of accuracy and reflect
the status of fundamental mechanisms with some reliability. For example, anthropometric measurements fall
in this category.

In other instances, such as the exact quantification
of nutritional status, a variety of sources of data such
as clinical, biochemical, dietary, etc., are needed and,
at best, do not absolutely describe the individual's

situation. Evaluation of behavior and performance is also a very complex undertaking with available methods being somewhat limited in their capacity to identify small variations from normal and in their lack of reliability before 4 to 5 years of age. Even then, it is impossible to be certain of the individual's long-term learning and behavioral capabilities.

Furthermore, there are major dimensions of study that are just beginning to be applied to the problem of malnutrition and brain function. These include more sophisticated techniques for electrophysiological measurement, determination of changes in the neuroendocrine systems, evaluation of neurotransmitter mechanisms such as the catecholamines, and greater quantification of sociological factors and their impact. Progress in future developments of these various techniques will undoubtedly help to expand our understanding of the mechanisms involved in these problems and help to facilitate their correction and prevention.

Finally, the importance of all of this is not only for advancement of our scientific knowledge, but for the development of a substantive base for social action. It is obvious that if all nutritional and environmental deficiencies could be eliminated, the problems they incur would disappear. However, such a Utopia is not forthcoming and so government policymakers and planners throughout the world are confronted with assessment of the nature and extent of their particular situation as well as with determination of the priorities for their solutions. The problems are different in various parts of the world and require selected measures for their solution. These will depend to a large extent on the findings from studies such as those that I have mentioned and others that must be undertaken in the near future.

CRITIQUE OF RESEARCH DEALING WITH THE CONSEQUENCES
OF EARLY MALNUTRITION

(Summary of discussion at the workshop on Nutrition)*

Participants: Drs. Bell, Berry, Collier, Coursin,
Cravioto, Pollitt, Stewart, Susser, Turkewitz,
Underwood, and Winick

The following summary of the participants' comments
regarding the experimental and clinical studies of infant malnourishment, while reflecting the major points
touched upon, does not provide the flavor of a lengthy,
intense and, at times, heated discussion of research
issues. While the participants could not reach agreement
upon some points, the editor's impressions were that most
left the discussion with some new information and an expressed need to re-examine their own research programs and
theoretical positions.

Most of the discussion focused upon the issue of the
mechanism(s) involved in the effects of malnourishment
upon growth and behavior. The major issues involved:
(a) can the effects of malnourishment be interpreted in
a straightforward organic-deficiency model, or must it
involve indirect mechanisms, e.g., modified interaction
with the environment; (b) the problems of definition and
measurement of organic versus functional mechanisms; and
(c) the role of task-demands in assessing the effects of
early malnutrition. The second portion of the discussion
consisted mostly of a description of "The Dutch Famine"
by its principal investigators (Dr. Mervyn Susser and his
wife, Dr. Zena Stein).

----

*Edited by Robert W. Bell

THE INTERPRETATION OF MALNOURISHMENT

Two opposing "strong" positions were initially
advocated. The first position posited a direct malnour-
ishment-deficient organic growth-behavioral deficits
model. That is, inadequate nutritional intake during
early life, when the organism is exhibiting rapid growth
and differentiation, results in selective and partial
failures in development. The developmental deficits are
measurable (at least potentially) at many levels of
analysis; e.g., anatomical, physiological, biochemical;
and are the basis of any detected behavioral deficits.

The opposing "strong" position posited an epigenetic,
or interactive, model. This position posited a mal-
nourishment-(deficient organic growth?)-reduced organ-
ism/environmental interaction-behavioral deficits model.
That is, building upon the experimental and theoretical
literature stemming from Hebb's neuropsychological
theory, the advocates of this strong position emphasized
the differential quality and quantity of early environmental stimulation experiences by the malnourished infant
when compared to the adequately nourished infant, with
most observed long-term consequences of malnourishment
attributable to these differences in early stimulation.

The ensuing discussion of these two beginning positions emphasized the following points:

1. Any attempt to dichotomize organic versus
functional causality is futile and, in fact, an archaic
distinction. Certainly, any long-term changes in behavior must be reflected at some level of biological
change; e.g., molecular, neurochemical, electrolytic;
and failure to find gross anatomical correlates does not
support a position which ignores organic bases of behavioral change.

2. Appeals to the published research and clinical
literature are not sufficient to settle the issues of
concern. During the formal paper presentations, several
investigators had reported interactive effects of experi-
mentally-manipulated environmental contingencies with
degrees of malnourishment. Further, Dr. Cravioto's
studies of "The Land of the White Dust" had suggested
some nonnutritional social factors which influenced the
effects of chronic malnourishment. However, the fact
that nonnutritional factors can modify the consequences
of early malnourishment does not provide a logical basis

for insisting that such factors must, of necessity, be
involved in any observed effects of early malnourishment.

3. Experimental studies of early malnourishment involving infrahuman animals exhibit a fair degree of
replicability (although not perfect). However, field
studies of malnourishment in humans sometimes find
long-term consequences and sometimes fail to detect any
measurable deficit. Since the experimental studies
characteristically are conducted under conditions of
environmental control, while the field studies, of
necessity, do not control for study-to-study variation
in environmental stimulation, it was suggested that the
interactive position was supported. However, several
considerations were raised which again caused a rejection
of this interpretation. First, the precision of measurement of organic (or behavioral) deficits is not great.
Second, the investigators may have selected inappropriate
indices in attempting to assess the effects of the malnourishment. Third, the task demands (especially true
for the field studies) may be such that in one society
(e.g., agrarian economy) considerable organic damage may
be undetectable in terms of behavioral (e.g., intellectual) functioning whereas the same degree of organic
deficit may result in inadequate functioning in a complex
technological society, in which intellectual demands upon
more individuals are relatively greater.

4. There was general agreement that the task of the
investigator of infant malnutrition remains the classic
task of the scientist. That is, he must replicate his
investigations of early malnourishment under a variety
of circumstances with a variety of organic and behavioral
endpoints in order to establish an empirical basis for
estimating the generality of his effects.

THE DUTCH FAMINE STUDY

The discussion group was fortunate to have Dr.
Mervyn Susser, the principal investigator of the Dutch
Famine Study, as one of their discussants. Dr. Susser
provided a brief description of his monumental study
of long-term consequences of a famine of limited duration.

The famine was clearly demarcated in time—6 months—
and place—western Holland—resulting from the systematic
destruction of food sources by the German Occupation Army.

The investigators selected two cities within the famine
area and sixteen "control" cities from outside the famine
area for their investigation. Since 97% of all citizens
were inducted into military service at 18 years of age,
the affected birth cohorts could be identified in terms
of prenatal exposure to the famine, and the specific
period and duration of exposure during gestation. Addi-
tionally, mortality data extending from birth to age of
induction were collected.

A total sample of 400,000 births were included in
the analyses of the sample. Of these, approximately half
were from the famine area; the remainder were from outside the famine area. Of those in the famine area about
25,000 were from cohorts which would have been exposed
to famine conditions during gestation. Thus, there are
simultaneous control cohorts from outside the famine
region and before-and-after cohort controls from within
the famine region. A specific sample of 6000 individuals
was identified, based upon birth in one of five teaching
hospitals, to estimate birth rate variation due to the
famine. There was a reduced birth rate. However,
analysis of the sample suggests that associated phenomena,
such as reduction in libido, caused the reduction in
fertility. There was no evidence of a selective absence
of the male population, e.g., which would show class
differences.

The cohorts exposed to the famine did show an elevated mortality which was restricted to the first 90 days
postparturition. The total elevation in mortality was
small and had minimal effects upon the other cohort comparisons, even with a working assumption that had they
survived they would have constituted those most severely
intellectually retarded.

Growth characteristics collected at birth indicate
that there were famine-related growth deficits. These
included such indices as head circumference and body
weight, with the famine-exposed cohorts ranging from 240
grams to 400 grams (about 16%) lighter than their cohort
controls.

Utilizing sample characteristics collected by the
military at the time of induction, cohort comparisons
were computed for all available characteristics. The
overall outcome was that the cohort samples showed
essentially no quantitative differences on virtually all
the measures. Specifically, the distribution of I.Q.

measures showed no famine-related effects, neither in
terms of mean values nor in terms of proportion of
extreme values. All additional indices of development,
either physical or behavioral, failed to discriminate
between the groups with a single exception. Dutch
psychiatrists use a categorical label of "immature
personality" to denote certain related characteristics.
A higher proportion of the famine-exposed cohort was so
labeled. The investigators are attempting to obtain a
specific set of descriptive characteristics which are
the basis for the "immature personality" syndrome to
better interpret the one long-term consequence of the
famine.

DISCUSSION

A number of discussants contrasted the Dutch
famine study with the studies which followed the siege
of Leningrad, which found marked effects of malnutrition
upon intellectual functioning as well as a number of
additional characteristics. It was pointed out that
the two situations were not comparable in that:

1. The Leningrad siege was prolonged over several
years, rather than being a sharply-demarcated event.

2. Leningrad residents were exposed to a number of
severe stresses, e.g., bombardment, severe cold, etc.,
that were not present during the Dutch famine.

3. The severity of malnutrition was greater, with a
characteristic difference in birth weight averaging 600
grams, in contrast with the 240 to 400 gram difference
in the Dutch study.

The author pointed out that the value of the Dutch
study lay in the unconfounding of malnutrition with the
kinds of nonnutritional variables which characteristically
accompany infantile malnutrition, e.g., socioeconomic
class, race, etc.

One discussant commented that the one discriminating
index, immature personality, might be of genuine interest.
J. McVey Hunt of the University of Illinois has noted that
ghetto children, by virtue of the person/room density in
which they live, have experienced more physical and social
stimulation than the typical middle-class child by the
beginning of school age (although less effective language

and behavior-control training). Such children appear
to operate under a higher level of arousal, displaying
heightened activity levels, restlessness, and short
attention span. These behaviors characteristically are
labeled as "immature" by the classroom teacher under the
conditions of quiet and discipline imposed by the classroom setting. It was suggested that the famine-cohort
of the Dutch study might have received compensatory
stimulation, e.g., holding, rocking, etc., from their
parents and that the "immature personality" label may
reflect this extrastimuation-induced heightened arousal.
It was noted that similar phenomena have been observed
in laboratory studies of infantile stimulation.

A final conclusion reached in the discussion of the
study was that the failure to find many consequences of
prenatal malnutrition in the study does not demonstrate
a lack of long-term consequences. While the Dutch
military were totally cooperative with the investigators,
the sorts of data available on these samples were, of
necessity, limited. A broader sampling of behaviors may
well have yielded differences due to the famine.

SUMMARY

Mervyn Susser

Chairman, Department of Epidemiology
Columbia University
New York, N.Y.

It is without forewarning that I give you my random thoughts on what we have been talking about, and the sample is unlikely to be representative or unbiased.

Essentially, I think we posed the problems of the nature of the studies presented on the interaction of the social environment with nutrition; these have produced some fascinating results, which we reiterated. We have an alternative position, however, identified with vigor by Dr. Winick. He held that it is necessary to ask specific questions which are aimed at nutrition itself, if the objective of our studies is indeed the **effects of nutrition, and not merely descriptive analysis of the development of children.**

Here I intervened myself on the topic of studies **that we, in Epidemiology at Columbia, are engaged in, one the Dutch famine, and another the Prenatal Project in Harlem. These two studies offer the possibility of isolating the nutritional variable, and of determining what the constraints on generalization are in each study.**

Dr. Cravioto developed the view that from the welter of descriptive studies, we have begun to identify those independent and dependent variables that are worth studying and relating to each other. Given that we have identified such variables, we may now proceed to try to develop causal models. These are causal models of

241

processes in society; nutrition is seen in social context as a potential factor in later development, including mental competence. Most agreed that we have reached the stage in research where it is possible to set up multivariate models for observational studies, on the one hand, and also to set up intervention models on the other. From these we can begin to identify and to specify what kinds of stimuli and what kinds of intervention would be useful at this point of time.

It was emphasized that we ought to be careful, also, in discriminating what kinds of dependent variables we measure. This problem deserves as much attention as the kinds of independent variables to be measured. We need to be clear in our minds whether we are looking at the organic level of impairment, or at the psychological level of function, or at the social level of role, and we need to discriminate carefully between all these different levels of the outcome of nutritional deprivation.

DISCUSSION ON MEGAVITAMINS

REPLY TO "NUTRITION AND PSYCHIATRIC ILLNESS"
BY SEYMOUR KETY *

Humphrey Osmond

Director, Bureau of Research in Neurology
and Psychiatry
New Jersey Neuropsychiatric Institute
Princeton, New Jersey

*Edited by Mr. John Osmundsen, Managing
Editor, MEDCOM, Inc.

Ironically I have never really viewed megavitamins
from the nutritional perspective way. I have looked
upon them as being a pharmacological instrument, because allowing for the way we introduced them, we did
not perceive them as being a nutritional factor at
that time, and perhaps I stayed rather sluggishly behind with this point of view. But I have a difficult
position because my formidable friend, Seymour Kety, has
presented some powerful points of view which I would
like to refute in detail, although I feel I am not competent to refute all of them. I do not mean to say I
think there are not people who are competent to do this,
but I am not competent to do so; and secondly, it would
be impossible, with so cogent and intelligent a critic,
to attempt this in a quarter of an hour.

I am going to attempt to raise certain rather important points about how the megavitamin theory evolved
because I think it is important to understand its
development. My interest in this, of course, started
as a commission. Ironically, I got involved in the
first double-blind trials in psychiatry, which at that
time was a strange innovation. It was undertaken with
the help of the Canadian government, and we were not the
first ones, of course, with this particular megavitamin
study. Megavitamins were used for experimentation in
other studies, and then we got on to this double-blind

245

concept. We designed and set up what was then an extremely taut and also very slow way of testing our
hypothesis. If you compare this with the original
testing of chlorpromazine, you will discover it was
far, far slower and more deliberate, and, in my opinion,
this was a grave mistake. However, no one listened to
me.

At that time it was perfectly all right in psychiatry to publish single studies without comparison groups;
I think the double-blind study came in about 1937. On
the whole, I believe they have been a fairly good innovation, but as Elliot Slater pointed out, they had
disadvantages, and I believe their greatest disadvantage
occurs when you are using a homogeneous population.

Now from a commission's point of view, you do not
begin trials of any sort without some evidence of clinical success, and we received that evidence with some
8 cases in early 1952. It was from that point that we
started this double- or really triple-blind trial, in
which there were two active groups and one nonactive
group, and these were followed up for two years, until
the end of 1953. The results were not ready until 1956,
at which time we published them.

Since the findings were so remarkable, we asked
consultants in Ottawa to design further studies, which
continued until 1960. Now during that time, it would
obviously have been quite improper for me not to have
treated some other people with these substances, since
we believed that people could only benefit from them.
As Dr. Wittenborn and others have pointed out, these
trials are unbelievably slow and difficult, and the
harder you try, the more effort, energy, and money seems
to be required. As economic support for our formal,
prospective trials, we accepted a great many people whom
we treated and subsequently followed for a period of
many years, resulting in the publication of these data,
which were gathered from a combination of these two
groups. One cannot call them carefully controlled
studies because they are comparison groups. You cannot
have a time-controlled study unless you can measure all
variables, and no one knows these in schizophrenia, although you can set up all kinds of standards. Our
original sample was diagnosed by others according to
Bleuler's criteria, which I now believe to be invalid.
But they met the criteria, anyway.

Now, just to touch on one or two points; first, John Harvey Mason was not responsible for the trans-methylation theory. He admitted this, in fact, himself. It was John **Smythies** who conceived the notion, seeing the relationship between the two factors. John Harvey Mason confirmed it. John **Smythies** and I were in a position to know if it was even feasible.

Let me comment on Seymour Kety's nice point regarding the epinephrine method of injection. I think it is important to realize--and I am sure he would agree--that though this is an interesting approach, it does not necessarily tell us very much about endogenous epinephrine. It may or it may not. I do not see how one could work it out exactly, but I think the labeled epinephrine has to, in fact, be processed in certain ways to get the active form we proposed. The other factor which we also have to bear in mind is that whatever the result, it was introduced in the periphery of the body. We do not know that this same process goes on in the brain, and I do not think that the brain studies at the moment really tell us very much one way or the other. Therefore, I do not think they can be fully supported.

There is one little semantic point which I think I must also raise with Dr. Kety: that is, the question of establishing a hypothesis, as it were, to the satisfaction of all. In reality, one initially establishes a hypothesis to the satisfaction of the hypothesis-maker. As to our hypothesis satisfying others' criteria, we presumably would have had to extract adrenochrome, and, unfortunately neither Abraham Hoffer nor I ever extracted this substance. It was synthesized instead.

Now that I have propounded this idea, I find it very regrettable that it has become a matter of such vigorous and sometimes rather embittered difference of opinion, but I think there is a reason for this. Our work on niacin was published for nearly **10 years; however,** it was hardly being used at all. Now this was very surprising. **We put forward a nonproprietary substance (nicotinic acid), unbelievably moderate in cost, with at least a possibility of helping the schizophrenic.** On the other hand, enterprises of a commercial nature have substances which they wish to sell, and you cannot expect them to advertise a nonproprietary substance. In fact they were very generous to us. Merck gave us huge

quantities of nicotinic acid. I do not want you to think
I am accusing the drug companies, but I simply say I did
not expect them to behave unnaturally.

Because I thought we were going to discuss the
nutritional aspects, which I think are very important,
I am going to examine the studies discussed here in
detail. I think the big study of nicotinic acid is
very remarkable and interesting. My objection, which
I gave at the time, was twofold. One part I think is
valid, the other is really a sort of personal quirk.
The valid one is that during 1966—67 I really did not
think that I would not have suggested that three grams
was enough. You may ask why. The answer is that the
schizophrenics in Saskatchewan in the early 1950's
were a different animal, for a perfectly good reason.
They had no prior access to phenothiazines. It was
not possible for them to go along to their general
practitioner and have a year or two of phenothiazines,
which are very beneficial in a way. Probably many
people get through their first attack of schizophrenia
today on phenothiazines. As you are no doubt aware, it
was a lot more difficult to do this on barbiturates,
simply because the patient is so groggy that his family
does not like him anymore.

In Saskatchewan at that time we were getting
schizophrenics who were really very newly ill. We did
not know this at the time, of course, because that was
how schizophrenia appeared. They were usually rather
wild, extremely unwell, and frequently being given
heavy doses of barbituates by people who were becoming
progressively more worried about them. If they were
unlucky, of course, they were receiving many of the
less pleasing barbituates and were being made quite ill.
That particular situation was altered over the years
and we think that we arrived at this quite empirically:
heavily sedated schizophrenics for some reason or other
need more niacin. I do not know why. Originally we
believed that we would not benefit people who had not
been ill more than a year. We discovered that they did
benefit largely by accident. That is, as we developed
our tests, we found many schizophrenics who had been
ill a long time who nevertheless appeared to be rather
like schizophrenics who had been ill only a short time.
Based on these findings it seemed reasonable to try
the preparation on them, and we reasonably expected that
it would take a longer time for an effect. In addition
to this, in our follow-up studies we found what we

interpreted as a protective effect of this over a much
longer period of time than we had previously supposed.
We reported this in 1962. I think this has become a
very unfortunate issue, which resulted in divergent
differences of opinion. I am sorry that it should have
resulted in such great clashes among people whose views
I respect and like, but that is the way in which this
particular game is played.

Now I think there is another important idea to bear
in mind--that is, this is still in a sense a relatively
short-term affair. The controversy is now less than
ten years old, and in this field ten years is a very
short time.

Let me illustrate by example. In 1754, James Lind
published his famous paper in which he demonstrated the
theory that orange or lemon juice cured scurvy. His
famous study is well worth reading. In 1776, a year no
doubt familiar to you, a chap called Cook did the second
half of his famous experiment in which he circumnavigated
the globe, and, using citrus juice, lost remarkably few
men to scurvy. I think he lost one or two compared with
about thirty in his previous voyage--a highly significant
study. The British navy adopted this procedure in 1794.
Lucky for them that they did, otherwise they could not
have blockaded very long in 1805. Afterward they cele-
brated this event, with their sailors acquiring the
reputation of "lime juicers" (instead of taking lemon and
orange juice, they consumed lime juice). The consequence
of this was that they lost two-thirds of the ascorbic
acids necessary to prevent scurvy. By 1840, Virker had
challenged the whole notion of deficiency diseases. He
pointed out this notion as an impossible phenomenon,
and affirmed that there could not be diseases of this
kind. This was a remarkable stand to maintain. Need-
less to say, this concept became very unpopular, and
by 1900 the idea of a deficiency disease disappeared.
It was subsequently replaced by the idea of ptomaine.
Scurvy was held to be due to ptomaine poisoning. The
result of this was that another British sailor, Sir
Robert Falcon-Scott, lost his life in 1911, with the
best scientific advice of the day. He carried no lemons
or oranges with him, though Shackleton, on a similar
expedition, did, and had no cases of scurvey in the
Antarctic region. Oddly enough, in 1911, Garland Hopkins
opened the first very unpopular biochemistry laboratory
at Guy's Hospital in London, and shortly after that
Casimir Funk produced the idea of vitamins.

As you can see there is a rather long span of time
involved, as well as a wide spectrum of concepts. Although I am disappointed at the difference of opinion
between Dr. Kety and myself, I am still not really sur-
prised. Still I do wish to take issue with Dr. Kety on
a point which he is perfectly justified to maintain as
a scientist, and a position he ought to take, but one
which, as a clinician, I cannot support. If there had
been no testimonials this would indeed be damaging
clinical evidence. From the point of view of scientists,
a testimonial is of no importance, but from the point of
view of a clinician, it is rather important, because it
relates to a different kind of world and a different kind
of proposition. The great difficulty is to fuse the two.
One of the greatest clinical scientists, Osler, pointed
out many years ago how very difficult and how uncertain
this is, and I sincerely hope that we will be able to
find out whether these things work or not.

Now to return for the last few minutes of my talk
to the nutrition concept, which I thought we had come
here to discuss and debate, I wish to emphasize two
interesting points. One is a by-product of this issue
of whether our particular views are right or wrong.

In northern Saskatchewan, a family doctor called
Glenn Green, who, believing that the Indian children
had learning difficulties, inquired, through the use of
our perceptual tests, about those childrens' responses
and perceptions. He then treated those who had abnormal
scores with nicotinic acid. As a result, many of them
began to learn quite well again. (They had been on very
peculiar diets.) Another group of Canadians who were in
a Hong Kong prison for a long time returned exception-
ally ill and stayed so for a period of 20 years; three
had beri-beri and also pellagra. Many of them have died
since. Six were put on large doses of megavitamins, and
those six men are well today. We can see their files
from the V.A. These mens' lives have been substantially
altered. When they cease their vitamin intake, they
become ill again. These men do not appear psychotic,
interestingly enough, but this evidence does suggest
that a change takes place in people who have had severe
beri-beri and pellagra. It is well known that the
recovery from pellagra does not occur simply by taking
ordinary doses of B-vitamins; also some people seem to
develop a vitamin dependency. So from the nutritional
point of view, in a large world there may be a lot of
people like the Indian children and the Canadian pris-
oners, and that might be worth looking for.

RESPONSE TO DR. OSMOND'S COMMENTS

Seymour S. Kety

Department of Psychiatry
Harvard Medical School
Director, Psychiatric Research Laboratories
Massachusetts General Hospital
Boston, Massachusetts

Dr. Osmond has taken issue with our tests of the adrenochrome hypothesis on the thesis that injected epinephrine may not behave like endogenous epinephrine and because our studies were made on blood and urine. However, the adrenochrome hypothesis postulated that circulating epinephrine released by the adrenal medulla was oxidized to adrenochrome. Injecting it into the blood would seem to be an appropriate test of the hypothesis. It is rather odd that Dr. Osmond should now discount studies based upon examination of blood and urine since he and Hoffer had earlier claimed that adrenochrome was present in the blood of schizophrenic patients and was excreted in their urine. Altschule, whom Hoffer cites in support of the hypothesis, found adrenochrome in urine.

Dr. Osmond expresses some distress at the lack of acceptance of megavitamin therapy by the scientific community in contrast to the widespread acceptance of the antipsychotic drugs. Two examples of such drugs which have become important parts of psychiatric treatment throughout the world are chlorpromazine and lithium. The beneficial effects of chlorpromazine on schizophrenic patients were first demonstrated about 1950, and within three to five years it was being used extensively in Europe and America. Lithium, a nonproprietary drug, was first used in the treatment of manic-depressive psychosis in 1949. Shortly thereafter, it was examined

in carefully controlled trials in Denmark, and within a
few years had become accepted treatment in Europe and
finally in America. Neither of these agents required
extravagant claims to the public, attacks on the
"psychiatric establishment," the creation of a separate
school of psychiatry or the publication of an autonomous
journal. Their acceptance was based upon their obvious
effects in clinical experience and the consistent finding
in controlled double-blind studies that they were significantly effective.

I might also add that the findings which Dr. Rosenberg describes in this volume of the effective use of
large doses of specific vitamins in correcting particular
neurological disorders and their carefully worked-out
biochemical underpinnings were rapidly accepted by the
scientific community. Res ipsa loquitur.

REMARKS ON THE USE OF MEGAVITAMINS IN THE TREATMENT

OF SCHIZOPHRENIA

Morris A. Lipton

Director, Biological Sciences Research Center
Department of Psychiatry
University of North Carolina
Chapel Hill, North Carolina
        and
Chairman, APA Task Force on Vitamins and
Psychiatry

I was interested in Dr. Osmond's opening statement
that he conceived of the vitamins which he uses in megadoses as pharmacological agents, not as nutrients. If this
is the case, it may be an error to link Dr. Hoffer and Dr.
Osmond on this point because despite their long association
they apparently disagree on the question of how niacin
works in the treatment of schizophrenia. As of a year ago,
Dr. Hoffer was writing about schizophrenia as a type of
cerebral pellagra and was clearly taking the position that
niacin in megadoses was a nutrient which overcame the
vitamin deficiency in the brain of schizophrenics. Whether
niacin in megadoses is a nutrient or a pharmacological
agent is a rather important issue. It should be clarified
because it is quite muddy in the literature. The two positions are really incompatible. A molecule of nicotinic
acid cannot simultaneously function as a vitamin and as a
methyl acceptor. The usual definition of a vitamin of the
B complex is that it is an essential nutrient because it
is converted into a coenzyme required for vital metabolic
reactions. When nicotinic acid becomes a coenzyme--that is,
nicotinamide-adenine-dinucleotide--it cannot be a methyl
acceptor, because the nitrogen of the pyridine ring is tied
in linkage with ribose. On the other hand, when it is
functioning as a methyl acceptor, it cannot be a vitamin
in the usual sense because it cannot become a coenzyme. So
we run into the curious semantic concept that sometimes a
vitamin is not a vitamin. Another way of dramatizing this
is to point out that at nutritional doses, nicotinic acid
and nicotinamide are identical in terms of vitamin potency.

They are equimolar nutritionally. However, in large
pharmacological megadoses, nicotinic acid generates a
cutaneous flush and lowers blood cholesterol. Nicotinamide will do neither. So, the property of lowering
cholesterol or making a flush is a pharmacological
property of nicotinic acid, which is quite independent
of its character as a vitamin, because the nicotinamide
will not do it. Obviously, in large doses the vitamins
do not function solely as vitamins.

Another point that needs clarification has to do with
a language that almost has the quality of advertising.
The terms "megavitamins" and "orthomolecular" are commonly
used. Everybody knows, "vitamins are good for you."
Therefore megavitamins are even better and can do no harm.
But if we now accept Dr. Osmond's position, that nicotinic
acid acts pharmacologically, it would be more proper to
call the treatment "methyl acceptor" therapy, and leave
the term vitamin out of it, because this property of nicotinic acid has nothing to do with the fact that it is a
vitamin. In fact, I would myself like to see some other
more effective methyl acceptors tried clinically, because
as Dr. Kety pointed out, nicotinamide or nicotinic acid is
not a very good one. There may be better ones. I do not
think the transmethylation hypothesis is by any means dead
and it deserves testing in therapeutic trials with better
methyl acceptors.

Equally, the term "orthomolecular," as employed in
clinical treatment, is a misnomer. I do not know what is
orthomolecular about electroconvulsive therapy, which is
commonly used in the treatment of the schizophrenic by the
megavitamin and orthomolecular proponents. In fact, as I
read their literature, it seems that all patients who go
into Phase 2 treatment, meaning that they do not respond
just to nicotinamide or nicotinic acid, will then be
treated with ECT. But this point is not emphasized in the
language of the proponents. Nor is there anything orthomolecular about the action of phenothiazines, and most
patients receiving megavitamins also receive these drugs.
I had earlier referred to the fact that orthomolecular
psychiatry today is really an add-on procedure. Everything which is used by conventional psychiatrists is used
by the orthomolecular psychiatrist, but then the vitamins,
in large quantities are also used. Not only is nicotinic
acid used, but just about every water-soluble vitamin there
is, plus one fat-soluble vitamin, along with hormones and
penicillamine, are all frequently added. The clinical and
laboratory criteria for what vitamins should be added for
any individual patient are never specified, but each pa-

tient apparently receives individualized treatment according to the judgment of the physician. This makes it virtually impossible to replicate the treatment in controlled clinical trials. When I want to get humorous about it, I say it is like replicating my mother's goulash. It is never quite the same thing twice, and while it may have more or less common ingredients, the quality and quantity will vary a good deal. This is, of course, one of the major problems involved in attempts at replication. This also explains why the attempts at replication, like Dr. Wittenborn's, or the extensive attempts that have been conducted by Drs. Ban and Lehmann in Canada, have dealt with one variable at a time. They have elected to try nicotinic acid because it was the first vitamin for which therapeutic claims were made, and because it remains the cornerstone of megavitamin theory. Their results have been consistently negative.

How have they been negative? There were claims made initially by the proponents of megavitamins that in some cases nicotinic acid was effective alone without the phenothiazines. As a matter of fact, there was a time when phenothiazines were castigated, and I think it was Dr. Hoffer who said substances less dangerous than these have been withdrawn from the market and that they ought not to be used. But now they are used routinely by orthomolecular psychiatrists. However, in the treatment of acute schizophrenics, a trial by Ban and Lehmann of nicotinic acid alone was simply useless. Patients could not be managed in that fashion. Then came the next trial of nicotinic acid as an adjunct to phenothiazines: Does niacin alter the quantity of phenothiazines required? There was a claim by the megavitamin proponents that it halved the quantity of phenothiazines or barbituates required for patient management. The Ban study indicates that, if anything, niacin increased the quantity of phenothiazines required, rather than cutting it in half. Does niacin alter duration of hospitalization? The Ban data indicated that it increases hospitalization time. It certainly does not decrease it as the proponents would have us believe. One can go down the list of the various experiments that have been done and all of these have been quite consistently negative. Now Dr. Wittenborn's experiment, which I am sure we will discuss again later, offers the first hint of positive effects offered by people who are not members of the megavitamin school. Dr. Wittenborn's responding patients were acutely psychotic but had excellent premorbid histories. They may not, therefore, have been truly schizophrenic. This raises the question of the need for accuracy of diagnosis in outcome studies of schizophrenia treatment.

I have examined the literature of the orthomolecular
psychiatrists diligently to determine the criteria they use
for the diagnosis. I have done this because when one gets
claims that 90% of acute schizophrenics will get well on
megavitamins, the question of what is really meant by
schizophrenia is crucial. This is particularly true when
the patients are divided into three groups, depending on
severity, duration, and response to the vitamins, and
treatment differs for each group. I have never been able
to find a statement as to how many of those 90% who get
well and stay well on megavitamins are Phase 1 patients.
Such patients are ambulatory, do not need hospitalization,
score high on the Hoffer-Osmond Diagnostic Battery, and may
have malvaria. Such patients respond to nicotinic acid. I
would submit, however, that these need not be schizophrenics in the first place. I was somewhat intrigued to find a
statement by one of their own advocates, which I will read
to you. "As I used the HOD test more extensively, it was
surprising to find that a number of neurotics and cases of
personality disorder had high perceptual scores, and some
had high total scores; these individuals did not appear
to be schizophrenics or to be pseudoneurotic schizophrenics.
They tended to be those who were almost constantly flooded
with adrenaline and who showed such vasomotor responses as
sweaty palms, palpitations, and tremor. Such patients did
respond well to 3 g of nicotinic acid added to their medication." This statement suggests that there is a group of
patients who I suppose would be typically classified as
neurotics and who may be called schizophrenics by the
megavitamin advocates. They respond to nicotinic acid.

For the "Phase 2 patients," as I said earlier, the
value of niacin gets very difficult to assess because of
the frequent use of electroconvulsive therapy (which is not
used commonly now by most psychiatrists in the treatment of
schizophrenia) along with the use of the other medications.
"Phase 3 patients get even more varied polypharmacy. This
makes the whole problem of replication extraordinarily difficult, but it also makes it impossible to select out the
crucial therapeutic ingredient without controlled clinical
trials.

There are two more points that I would like to make.
Dr. Kety has already raised the first one; it is the issue
of credibility. Despite the fact that Dr. Osmond tells us
now that he really believes primarily in the pharmacological action of nicotinic acid, he was a co-author of that
most dramatic of all papers in the megavitamin therapy of
schizophrenia. I am referring to the one dealing with the
administration of the coenzyme NAD, nicotinamide-adenine-

dinucleotide. And that truly was a dramatic paper. I shall describe the results to you briefly. It said that patients who had been chronically ill for $9\frac{1}{2}$ years and were then given 1 g/day of the coenzyme (NAD) became well within 3 days. In the Table of Results there is an asterisk on top of the category "well." The footnote defines "well" as "gainfully employed, adjusted in the community, and getting along with their families." This degree of recovery occurred in $3\frac{1}{2}$ days. Well, such dramatic results strain credibility. It takes longer than 3 days to find a job if one has been ill for 9 years. It is also incredible because there is reason to believe that NAD, as an intact molecule, does not penetrate cells; so on biochemical grounds it is difficult to accept. Nonetheless, in contrast to what I feel was somewhat shameful treatment of the early papers of Hoffer and Osmond on nicotinic acid, which were essentially ignored for 10 years, this one was not ignored for very long. As I recall, within 30 days the first attempt at replication was started. Altogether there were four attempts made by independent investigators. Nathan Kline was the first to try. He was followed by Meltzer, Gallant, and others. Each one of these obtained negative results. Returning to the matter of credibility, when something as dramatic as the NAD results are claimed and immediately found wanting, then one automatically suspects other claims as well. The credibility of the megavitamin group was certainly very much damaged by this. I should emphasize, however, that the failure to replicate the NAD story does not in itself invalidate the nicotinic acid work, because nicotinic acid could conceivably be working by some mechanism other than NAD. At any rate, we have not heard anything about NAD since approximately 1968, and claims about its therapeutic value are simply not made any longer.

There is an additional reason to doubt the megavitamin claims. Remember, it is claimed that the results from nicotinic acid are better than those from the phenothiazines. These statements are supported by minimizing the results from phenothiazines and perhaps making the niacin data look better than they really are. There are other data that would indicate that the phenothiazine results, when carefully examined, as they have been by Goldberg, Fogarty, and Schooler, are better than those referred to by the orthomolecular psychiatrists. These are virtually as good as the results that are generally claimed by the megavitamin advocates.

I think that there is reason to be concerned about the way megavitamin proponents have castigated psychiatry in

the lay press, the megavitamin books, and their own Journal.
They have generated myths--the myth is still perpetuated
that most psychiatrists mistreat their schizophrenic patients by insisting upon doing intensive psychotherapy or
psychoanalysis with them, and that they do not employ
somatic treatments. The fact of the matter is that virtually no psychiatrists deal with schizophrenics without
using the phenothiazines or similar drugs at this time.
There may be a few psychotherapists who do this, but it
is a myth that most schizophrenics receive intensive
psychotherapy or psychoanalysis alone.

May I take the last minute by saying that I was
assigned the task of reviewing the megavitamin research
by the American Psychiatric Association because I have a
Ph.D. in Biochemistry. It also happens that I was a
graduate student at Wisconsin at the time when nicotinic
acid was discovered in their biochemistry department. I
was not lucky enough to be working on nicotinic acid--I
was working on thiamin--perhaps that kept me from being
famous; but I began with an initial prejudice, that indeed
there might be something that could be useful and dramatic
in the nicotinic acid treatment of schizophrenia. I examined the literature carefully, and aside from the little
clue that Dick Wittenborn has given us this morning, I
find nothing persuasive in the literature to indicate that
this is an effective treatment for even a minority of patients. There is no laboratory evidence to support the
theory. There is little empirical evidence to support the
therapeutic claims. There are some intriguing new findings
in clinical genetics that may or may not be relevant. I
trust that Dr. Rosenberg will talk about these. They deal
with the so-called vitamin-dependency illnesses. The
findings here are extremely impressive. But the vitamin-
dependency illnesses are quite different from schizophrenia, as I am sure he will point out. Other forms of
nutritional treatment may turn out to have value, but the
burden of proof is on the advocates, and they must perform
adequately controlled trials and present their data in
scientific journals before the scientific and clinical
community can accept them.

ACKNOWLEDGMENTS

Funded in part by Grant HD-03110 from the National
Institute of Child Health and Human Development.

CONTRAST BETWEEN VITAMIN-RESPONSIVE INHERITED METABOLIC DISEASES AND VITAMIN USE IN SCHIZOPHRENIA

Leon E. Rosenberg

Chairman, Department of Human Genetics
Yale University School of Medicine
New Haven, Connecticut

I am not a psychiatrist. I am an internist and a medical geneticist who has become interested in the question of the use of large doses of vitamins in the therapy of schizophrenia because of my involvement with a number of inherited metabolic diseases which I would like to tell you about briefly. In 1954, Hunt and his colleagues described two female siblings with neonatal convulsions whose seizure disorder was not controlled by the usually prescribed anticonvulsants or by physiologic doses of pyridoxine. When these girls were given 10 to 20 times the physiologic requirement, however, seizures stopped abruptly and recurred only after cessation of the pyridoxine supplements. This pattern of seizure control by large amounts of pyridoxine followed by exacerbation after vitamin withdrawal led Hunt to propose that these children were "dependent" on increased amounts of pyridoxine to prevent central nervous system hyperactivity. Thus, the concept of vitamin-dependent metabolic disorders was born. It is interesting, I think, to note that Hunt's study was reported at about the same time that Dr. Osmond first suggested that nicotinic acid was beneficial in schizophrenia. Since these early observations, the two fields of "vitamin-responsive" or "vitamin-dependent" inborn metabolic disorders and so-called "megavitamin-responsive" schizophrenia have followed very divergent courses. I shall underscore this divergence by first summarizing the pattern of investigation followed in the vitamin-responsive inborn errors of metabolism.

We now recognize more than 20 well-defined inborn
errors which respond dramatically, either clinically or
biochemically, to the administration of anywhere from 5
to 1000 times the usual physiologic dose of a specific
vitamin. These vitamin-responsive disorders are diverse
in clinical findings, biochemical abnormalities and
qualitative and quantitative vitamin requirement. For
example, in addition to pyridoxine-dependent seizures,
there are 5 other disorders which respond to large doses
of pyridoxine. Similarly, there are vitamin responsive
disorders which respond to thiamine, vitamin B12, folic
acid, biotin, and nicotinamide. Each of these disorders
is distinct from the other, and most are known to be due
to specific enzymatic abnormalities which have been defined by biochemical and genetic studies in vivo and in
vitro. The description of such conditions provides com-
pelling data to support the idea that a small number of
individuals in our society have requirements for a specific vitamin which are very different from that of the
general population. This concept, of course, is one of
the keystones of the orthomolecular psychiatry approach,
and appeared considerably earlier than Dr. Pauling's
formal statement concerning the latter notion.

Let me now contrast the scientific and clinical
evidence concerning these vitamin-responsive inborn
errors with that which exists for the use of large doses
of vitamins in schizophrenia. I shall refrain from using
the word "megavitamin" because it has a flamboyance and
military connotation which I dislike. First, let us consider the evidence for a genetic etiology. Each one of
the vitamin-responsive metabolic disorders has a clear
Mendelian mode of inheritance which identifies it as a
single gene abnormality. I believe we would all agree
that, whereas there is considerable evidence that genetic
factors may be important in the etiology of schizophrenia,
there is no convincing evidence for a monogenic hypothesis
of causation. Second, for virtually all of the known
vitamin-responsive inherited disorders, the specific
biochemical basis for the disorder is clear. This may
involve accumulation of substrates or metabolites in
blood and urine, or evidence of discrete enzymatic abnormality in tissues. In contrast, there is no clear-cut
biochemical basis for the disease constellation which is
given the name schizophrenia. Third, the use of a particular vitamin in the vitamin-responsive inborn errors
is based on a biochemical understanding of the disorder.
Thus, children with pyridoxine-dependent seizures have
a specific defect in the enzyme, glutamic acid decarbox-

ylase, which is known to be a pyridoxal phosphate-
dependent enzyme. Similarly, individuals with pyridox-
ine-responsive homocystinuria have an inherited deficiency in the pyridoxal phosphate-dependent enzyme,
cystathionine synthase. In each case there is a correlation between the particular biochemical defect
identified and the rationale for the specific vitamin
which has proven to be effective. No such rationale
exists at the present time for the use of large amounts
of many different vitamins in schizophrenia. Fourth,
the age of onset of the known vitamin-responsive inborn
errors is generally in infancy or early childhood. This,
of course, is not true for schizophrenia. Fifth, the
rapidity of remission and exacerbation following institu-
tion or cessation of vitamin therapy is quite different
in the vitamin-responsive metabolic diseases and in
schizophrenia. It has been amply demonstrated that with
the vitamin-responsive inborn errors biochemical manifestations or clinical changes occur within minutes,
hours or days. In no case has it taken months or years
to demonstrate improvement as has been stated for vitamin
effects in schizophrenia.

It may even be more pertinent to point out the only
known example of vitamin-responsive schizophrenia.
Recently, Freeman and his colleagues described a teen-
age boy with hallucinations, delusions, catatonia and
withdrawal unresponsive to psychotherapy. This patient
was found to have a specific defect in folic acid
metabolism and responded dramatically to folate supplements. A single vitamin was sufficient, response was
rapid, and a biochemical basis was at hand.

As a clinician, I can understand the forces which
drive clinicians or investigators to use any potentially
effective form of therapy in schizophrenia. The vitamin-
responsive inborn errors of metabolism which I have been
discussing affect very few patients. They are each a
rare experiment of nature, significant to a handful of
people, whereas schizophrenia is a major health problem
and, therefore, attracts to it a very different socio-
logic urgency. I understand this sense of urgency and
think a strong case can be made for the controlled
administration of large amounts of multiple vitamins for
a short period of time in patients with newly diagnosed
schizophrenia. If dramatic changes are observed, intense
investigation may then be conducted to determine which
vitamin is effective. This is a very different format
from that currently recommended by the proponents of
vitamin therapy in schizophrenia.

Finally, let me point out, that as Dr. Wittenborn's study so clearly indicates, we can never assume that because 5 mg of nicotinic acid or pyridoxine or vitamin B12 is innocuous, it therefore follows that 500 mg or 5000 mg is equally harmless. Some patients with homocystinuria have been shown to develop seizures when they were treated with huge doses of pyridoxine. The hyperpigmentation that Dr. Wittenborn observed in some of his patients has been documented in others receiving huge amounts of nicotinic acid. We all know that the administration of such fat-soluble vitamins as vitamins A and D in large amounts can produce serious and even lethal consequences. Surely the credo of a physician to do no harm must apply as equally to the therapy of schizophrenia as it does to the treatment of any illness in a child or adult.

REFERENCES

Freeman, J. M., Finkelstein, J. D., Mudd, S. H., and Uhlendorf, B. W., 1972, "Homocystinuria presenting as reversible schizophrenia--a new defect in menthionine metabolism and reduced methylene-tetrahydrofolate-reductase activity," Pediat. Res. 6:163 (abstract).

Hunt, A. D. Jr., Stokes, J. Jr., McCrory, W. W., and Stroud, H. H., 1954, "Pyridoxine dependency: Report of a case of intractable convulsions in an infant controlled by pyridoxine," Pediatrics, 13:140-145.

Mudd, S. H., Uhlendorf, B. W., Freeman, J. M., Finkelstein, J. D., and Shih, V. E., 1972, "Homocystinuria associated with decreased methylenetetrahydrofolate reductase activity," Biochem. Biophys. Res. Commun 46:905-912.

Rosenberg, L. E., 1973, "Vitamin dependent genetic disease," in: Medical Genetics (V. A. McKusick and R. Claiborne, eds.) pp. 73-79, H. P. Press, New York.

Scriver, C. R., and Rosenberg, L. E., 1973, "Vitamin-responsive aminoacidopathies," in: Amino Acid Metabolism and Its Disorders, pp. 453-478, Saunders, Philadelphia.

Scriver, C. R., and Whelan, D. T., 1969, "Glutamic acid decarboxylase (GAD) in mammalian tissue outside the central nervous system, and its possible relevance to hereditary vitamin B6 dependency with seizures," Ann. N.Y. Acad. Sci. 166:83-96.

Yoshida, T., Tada, K., and Arakawa, T., 1971, "Vitamin B6 dependency of glutamic acid decarboxylase in the kidney from a patient with vitamin B6-dependent convulsion," Tohoku J. Exp. Med. 104:195-198.

THE TRANSMETHYLATION HYPOTHESIS RESTATED

Arnold J. Friedhoff

Director, Millhauser Laboratories
New York University School of Medicine
New York, N.Y.

I want to briefly discuss the transmethylation
hypothesis and try to restate it in a way that will
incorporate some more recent findings. There appears
to be considerably greater support for this hypothesis
from recent biochemical and pharmacological findings
than from therapeutic tests involving the administration
of nicotinic acid and nicotinamide. When Harley-Mason,
Smythies, and Osmond proposed the transmethylation
hypothesis, they were concerned principally with the
possibility that epinephrine might be methylated to an
analog of mescaline or to a hallucinogenic molecule.
More recently a number of investigations have been
concerned with the role of dopamine, rather than epinephrine, in psychosis, and the possible involvement of
methylated derivatives of dopamine. This change in
interest has occurred largely because of the discovery
that a decrement in dopaminergic activity is responsible
for the pathology in both drug-induced and naturally
occurring Parkinsonism.

It has now been well established that all effective
antipsychotic drugs can produce Parkinsonian symptoms.
Furthermore, it has been observed more recently, that all
anti-Parkinson's drugs, regardless of their chemical
classification, have the potential for producing psychosis. It has also been shown that antipsychotic drugs of
several types block the action of dopamine through several mechanisms. From these observations, a number of
investigators have concluded that the antidopaminergic

action of antipsychotic drugs, which results in
Parkinsonism in high dose, may be the mechanism by
which they produce some of their therapeutic effects.
One conclusion that can be derived from those observations is that an excess of dopaminergic activity may
be involved in the pathogenesis of at least some of the
**symptoms of psychosis. In other words, if the effects
of dopamine are decreased by antipsychotic drugs and
therapeutic benefit results, then perhaps dopamine
itself is involved in the pathogenesis of some of the
symptoms that disappear in response to anti-psychotic
drug treatment.**

Since the time this hypothesis was first proposed,
a number of investigators have developed considerable
evidence which indicates that dopamine probably is in
some way, central to the pathogenesis of certain symptoms
of psychosis. It is also our view that the dopaminergic
system may be implicated in the pathogenesis of certain
symptoms of psychosis, but may not necessarily be the
**locus of the primary etiological process (Friedhoff and
Alpert, 1973). Etiology and pathogenesis in schizo-**
phrenia should be considered separately. In the case of
amphetamine psychosis, for instance, we have known for
years that the etiological agent is amphetamine. Until
recently, this has not been very helpful in understanding the pathogenesis of this psychosis.

At this point in the development of the biochemistry
of mental illness, we are interested not only in primary
etiological factors, since we often have very little clue
as to what they are, but also in understanding the
mechanisms that are involved in the formation of symptoms.
In the case of dopamine, we can begin to consider the
symptoms that are relieved by antipsychotic drugs, all
of which decrease dopaminergic activity in the central
**nervous system by one mechanism or another. The
dopamine hypothesis does not incorporate all of the**
available empirical data. However, this hypothesis does
permit the integration of a large number of findings
from several disciplines.

Major support for the notion that dopamine is
central in the production of some of the symptoms of
psychosis have come from studies of Snyder et al. (1970),
who has made a strong case for the fact that certain of
the behavioral effects in amphetamine psychosis appear
to be related to the hyperdopaminergic effect of amphetamine, whereas the arousal effects appear to result from

the hyperadrenergic effects. This proposal has been directly tested in humans by Angrist et al. (1971), and the findings support Snyder's proposal.

Recently we have demonstrated that there is an enzyme present in mammalian liver and brain which is capable of converting dopamine to a di-O-methyl derivative which behaves like a hallucinogen in animals (Friedhoff et al., 1972). We have also shown that a pathway exists for the conversion of dopamine to mescaline. Mammalian tissues are capable of producing mescaline. This enzyme may simply be adventitious and may reflect nothing much more than that we are in some way relatives of the peyote cactus, the principle source of mescaline. On the other hand, it may reflect the fact that hallucinogenic molecules, which can be synthesized by normal mammalian tissues, may have some normal function which is disturbed in patients who are psychotic. The conversion of dopamine to mescaline or to the other hallucinogenic derivatives involves transmethylation, in that methyl groups are transferred from S-adenosylmethonine to dopamine or a methoxylated derivative of dopamine. Axelrod (1961) has shown that serotonin or tryptamine can be converted respectively to bufotenin and dimethyltryptamine (DMT), also through the transfer of a methyl group. DMT is a potent hallucinogen. Bufotenin crosses the blood-brain barrier poorly, but is also probably hallucinogenic when it enters the brain.

In view of these findings we must begin to determine whether these endogenous hallucinogenic molecules have any normal physiological functions, what those might be, and whether they are in any way involved as mediators of some of the symptoms of psychotic reactions.

REFERENCES

Angrist, B. M., Shopsin, B., and Gershon, S., 1971, "Comparative psychotomimetic effects of stereoisomers of amphetamine," Nature 234:152.

Axelrod, J., 1961, "Enzymatic formation of psychotomimetic metabolites from normally occurring compounds," Science 134:343.

Friedhoff, A. J., and Alpert, M., 1973, "A dopaminergic-cholinergic mechanism in production of psychotic symptoms," Biol. Psychiatr. 6:165.

Friedhoff, A. J., Schweitzer, J. W., and Miller, J.,
    1972, "The enzymatic formation of 3,4-Di-O-methylated
    dopamine metabolites by mammalian tissues," Res.
    Commun. Chem. Pathol. Pharmol. 3:293.
Snyder, S. H., Taylor, K. M., Coyle, J. T., and
    Meyerhoff, J. L., 1970, "The role of brain dopamines
    in behavioral regulation and actions of psychotropic
    drugs," Am. J. Psychiatr. 127:117.

SUMMARY

Morris A. Lipton

Director, Biological Sciences Research Center
Department of Psychiatry
University of North Carolina
Chapel Hill, North Carolina
     and
Chairman, APA Task Force on Vitamins and
Psychiatry

The megavitamin discussion was characterized, I think,
by lack of data on the part of the proponents. Nonetheless, case reports and strongly positive opinions were
offered.

Dr. Osmond, who was the first speaker, addressed
himself essentially to a pharmacological action of large
doses of niacin in the treatment of schizophrenia and gave
us a detailed discourse on the history of the development
of the concept. In the course of this history he did point
out an interesting phenomenon: they had been making their
claims for ten years before anyone paid attention, even to
deny them; and this, it seems to me, is perhaps the worst
fate that can befall any scientist. It does lead, I think,
as it did, to going to the lay press and to making somewhat extravagant statements. This may account for some of
the irresponsible actions of the proponents of megavitamin
therapy.

The remainder of the discussion, which Leon Rosenberg,
Dr. Friedhoff, and I, and then speakers from the floor
pursued, was basically quite critical of the whole concept
of megavitamins and their usefulness in schizophrenia.
For that reason I think it might be quite proper for me
to curtail my time and to give some of it to Dr. Osmond
so that he might have the opportunity to reply to some of
the questions that have been raised about this theory and
practice of megavitamin therapy.

In my presentation, I pointed out some of the con-
ceptual inconsistencies which occur in the hypothesis regarding the utility of niacin in schizophrenia. I referred
to the many types of data that have been negative, and
that have failed to replicate the results of the proponents.
I also pointed out the difficulties in replicating a therapeutic program that has so many variables. These include
everything from cereal-free diets to hormones, vitamins,
and psychotropic drugs simultaneously. Even though it is
not usually presented in this fashion, the fact of the
matter is that what is called megavitamin therapy is always
an adjunctive therapy, added on to the types of treatments
that all other psychiatrists use. It is not a substitute
treatment. It is not used instead of phenothiazines or
butyrophenones. There is perhaps one significant difference between what megavitamin therapists and conventional psychiatrists do. I am under the impression that
electroconvulsive therapy is used a good deal more by the
megavitamin people. It is possible, but not likely, that
this could make a difference in the effectiveness of the
megavitamins.

I was then followed by Leon Rosenberg, who gave a
very elegant presentation of the nature of the vitamin-
dependency illnesses with which he has worked. There are
now 15 of these, implicating most of the water-soluble
vitamins. Those of you who listened carefully may recall
that he listed every B complex vitamin except nicotinic
acid. There are vitamin-dependency illnesses for thiamine,
folic acid, B_6, biotin, and riboflavin, but there are as
yet none for nicotinic acid. This leaves me with the
whimsical feeling that perhaps the megavitamin people
picked the wrong vitamin to start with. It is conceivable
that their idea may be sound, but the wrong vitamin was
chosen and for the wrong reasons.

Dr. Rosenberg, also emphasized the differences between the vitamin-dependency illnesses and schizophrenia.
The former are characterized by the fact that they are
Mendelian in genetic inheritance; they are demonstrated
early in life--that is, in infancy or very early in childhood; they invariably have biochemical correlates; they
have quite specific clinical features; and they respond
dramatically, from within hours to perhaps one or two days,
to the replacement by large doses of vitamins. Such doses
would ordinarily be called pharmacological because they
are twenty to several hundred times the ordinary dose, but
for patients with such illnesses these doses are physiological. But the vitamin-dependency illness, as has been

pointed out, appear to be quite different from adult schizophrenia.

Dr. Friedhoff then spoke of the transmethylation hypothesis, and I think most of us would agree with him that this is not yet dead and may be correct. However, it still needs testing. The nicotinic acid therapeutic test is far from an adequate one.

Now, if I may take one or two moments more, there are a couple of thoughts that I have that did not come up in the discussion. The first is that it does seem to me that this kind of argument or debate is frequent, and perhaps inevitable, with most common, serious, and chronic illnesses. Obviously, there is much room for development in the treatment of schizophrenia. I have no doubt that until we have a great deal more understanding and more effective treatment, many unsubstantiated claims will be made.

Due to the early emphasis of a decade or more ago on the total psychogenesis of schizophrenia, which most of us would no longer accept, there has been enormous guilt on the part of parents, because they feel responsible for the schizophrenia of their children. Therefore, many of them welcome the idea that their child has a metabolic disease. I have no doubt that, right or wrong, one of the attractions of those who have espoused the megavitamin concept is that it does indeed reduce guilt on the part of parents and relatives and also shame on the part of parents and and relatives and also shame on the part of the individuals who have the illness. It is now no worse, if you like, to have schizophrenia than it might be to have diabetes, gout, or something similar. That has in itself had socially useful spinoffs, like the formation of Schizophrenics Anonymous and other self-help organizations. This is all countered by the fact that, as Dr. Mosher pointed out, a wrong concept and inadequate treatment can also have fairly devastating effects. If the treatment is not effective, and we have all encountered cases where people have come to us following failures in megavitamin therapy, then there is total despair on the part of the patients and the relatives.

The last thought is one that I really owe to Dr. Kety from an earlier discussion. Claims of the utility of the megavitamins are by no means limited to schizophrenia. They include childhood autism, alcoholism, arthritis, hypercholesterolemia, addiction, and some forms of

senility. Perhaps that is as it should be, because in
reviewing the literature on pellegra some months ago, I
did find that pellagra does indeed manifest itself in
many ways. Depending upon the age of the patient, the
severity of the illness, and its chronicity, it can
manifest itself as neurasthenia, depression, or florid
organic psychosis. Furthermore, there is indeed apparently such a phenomenon as pellagra sine pellagra; that
is, without the manifestations of the skin lesions, the
glossitis, and the diarrhea. It does not happen often,
but it does occur occasionally.

And so if niacin has any utility at all in megavitamin quantities, it might be useful for illnesses
other than schizophrenia. The possibility is remote, but
it might function as a vitamin or coenzyme for an iso-
steric enzyme with a different dissociation constant.
Perhaps forms of vitamin-dependency illness will be found
for nicotinic acid, but only future research will determine that. The question of the utility of meganicotinic
acid treatment for schizophrenia is moribund for most
critical investigators. There was no evidence presented
that would persuade us that meganiacin therapy has any
utility. Quite recently, I saw a copy of a book we have
all been waiting for for about two years. This book is
called Orthomolecular Psychiatry, edited by Linus Pauling
and David Hawkins. To show that I am totally fair, may
I plug it? I at least will read it, in the hope that
there will be information there that is not yet available
to us, and that might conceivably be more persuasive than
that which has been given to us at this time.

COMMENT

Humphrey Osmond

Director, Bureau of Research in Neurology
and Psychiatry
New Jersey Neuropsychiatric Institute
Princeton, New Jersey

First I would like to say that I am commenting not because I in any way believe that Dr. Lipton has not fairly summarized the discourse. I am sure he has done that very well. I will end simply on this note: The **problem that one faces in this particular kind of investigation is that it is absolutely impossible, unless you produce a very different form of design, ever to see a patient getting well in these circumstances;** unless you break the double-blind concept, you will never know. This phenomenon in medicine impresses one, perhaps erroneously; when you cannot see all variables in these double-blind studies, you tend to have a somewhat different opinion. This is how the opinion developed, having tested it clinically, using the methods which the methodologist believe work, and which, as Elliott Slater pointed out, have never yet contributed to any discovery in medicine. Slater said this about two years ago. So, I leave you commending these methods. I hope the methodologists will improve them, but, as a clinician, my pleasure has been to see people who, I believe--perhaps erroneously--improved in these circumstances. In the long run, I am afraid it is history that will judge us all.

CONCLUSIONS AND INDEX

CLOSING REMARKS

George Serban

**Medical Director, Kittay Scientific Foundation
        and**
New York University Medical Center
New York, N.Y.

Distinguished scientists and members of the press,
on behalf of the Kittay Scientific Foundation, I warmly
thank you for your dedicated and articulate partici-
pation, which has brought clarification to important
issues in the field of nutrition and biochemistry of
mental illness, advancing and integrating knowledge in
the field of psychiatry.

Your highly scientific and original presentation,
your engaging and critical discussion during the work-
shops, have created the basis for a free academic interaction and a truly scientific exchange of ideas.

I hope that the creative spirit which has dominated
the entire period of the symposium will be translated
into productive research in your laboratories and extended into your work in the field. The issues are
complex and challenging. **They have been confronted**
intelligently and skillfully. Through your quality of
validating research, you are contributing quietly but
forcefully towards the shaping of some future aspect of
society. To the extent to which your findings belong to
the field of public health, your scientific data will
constitute the basis for formulating social policies for
economics, governmental agencies, and public health
services.

The Kittay Scientific Foundation, socially conscious
and concerned with epidemiological aspects of nutrition,
inaugurated this series of symposia on malnutrition in

275

order to stimulate high quality research in the field.
The Foundation has decided to introduce the Kittay
International Award of $25,000 in next year's psychiatric,
scientific competition, in which the area of nutrition
will also be included. If the subject of nutrition is
designated as the final choice by the International Advisory Board, the award will be offered to the most
distinguished scientist whose contribution was responsible for a major impact on the understanding and treatment of the problem of malnutrition.

Once again, allow me to express my pleasure in the
unqualified success of this symposium and thank you for
your dedicated work and enthusiasm.

INDEX